NOTES FOR THE ACADEMIC CLINICIAN

M000187973

NOTES FOR THE ACADEMIC CLINICIAN

Stephen A. Geraci, M.D.
and
Mary Jane Burton, M.D.

with Foreword by G. Richard Olds, M.D.
and Introduction by S. Calvin Thigpen, M.D.

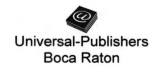
Universal-Publishers
Boca Raton

Notes for the Academic Clinician

Copyright © 2012 Stephen A. Geraci
All rights reserved.
No part of this book may be reproduced or transmitted in
any form or by any means, electronic or mechanical,
including photocopying, recording, or by any information
storage and retrieval system, without written permission
from the publisher

Universal-Publishers
Boca Raton, Florida • USA
2012

ISBN-10: 1-61233-082-7
ISBN-13: 978-1-61233-082-2

www.universal-publishers.com

Cover photo © Bocanm | Dreamstime.com

Library of Congress Cataloging-in-Publication Data

Geraci, Stephen A., 1957-
  Notes for the academic clinician / Stephen A. Geraci, Mary
Jane Burton.
      p. ; cm.
  Includes bibliographical references.
  ISBN 978-1-61233-082-2 (pbk. : alk. paper) -- ISBN 1-
61233-082-7 (pbk. : alk. paper)
  I. Burton, Mary Jane, 1971- II. Title.
  [DNLM: 1. Faculty, Medical. 2. Vocational Guidance. W
21]

  610.23--dc23

                                        2011050058

DISCLAIMER

The ideas, suggestions, advice and recommendations contained in this book are solely those of the authors, and do not represent the opinions, policies or positions of the publisher, the University of Mississippi, or any other group or entity. This content is intended to raise awareness of issues related to aspects of physicians' professional activities in academic clinical medicine, and to suggest techniques to improve productivity and job satisfaction, along with possible solutions for common problems encountered in such a career. This book should be viewed as a general guide and not professional advice on what to do in the reader's specific situation. No guarantee whatsoever is made to suggest that the contents of this book represent definitive plans or actions that will be optimal, or effective, in all circumstances. Readers are urged to examine their particular situations, seek out guidance from known, trusted advisors and other resources, and act based upon their own analysis of their professional situation in ways that will best achieve their desired results.

DEDICATIONS

For this book, I must make two dedications to recognize those who provided me the knowledge and ability to reach the career stage to write this collection.

The first dedication is to the students, residents, fellows and junior faculty members whom I have trained and mentored over the last three decades. It has been an uncommon privilege to work with such bright, dedicated young people, and to watch with pride as they succeeded in all fields of health care, teaching and academics. I have learned much through our relationships, and their achievements continue to provide my own greatest career satisfaction.

However, this book is only a small piece of a 35-year career (to date) that has consumed innumerable hours and regularly left me exhausted, sometimes frustrated, and with little time or energy remaining to attend to all the needs of personal life and family. So the single greatest effort for this book, by providing the support that allowed me to live the life and gain the experiences upon which this book is based, has been from my wife Terry—the absolute love of my life, my best friend, my strength and my comfort, for more than a quarter century. Her devotion, caring, and commitment leaves me without words adequate to express my gratitude. This book is truly hers.

-SG

ACKNOWLEDGEMENTS

I am most grateful to Janice Swinton, an accomplished author and editor in her own right, for her invaluable efforts in preparing this manuscript and helping launch our faculty development program in the Department of Medicine of the University of Mississippi. Janice encouraged the initial concept of converting a group of advice papers into a book, and did much of the work needed to bring this project to publication. There would be no "Notes for the Academic Clinician" without her commitment.

I also thank Sue Downey for the copy editing, and for turning my script into appropriate printed English. Sue is a gifted professional and kindred spirit in the world of medical scholarship.

Thanks also go to G. Richard Olds, M.D., my friend for many years and the most forward thinker I have met during my professional life.

Finally, I thank my supporting author, Mary Jane Burton, M.D., and the writer of the Introduction, S. Calvin Thigpen, M.D., who provided topic ideas, advice, content, feedback and honest criticism throughout the development of this work. They are among the best examples I know of why we must teach and mentor: our junior colleagues are both the rewards of our efforts, and the future of our profession.

-SG

CONTENTS

Foreword

Over the years I have held many senior leadership positions in academic medicine, including division chief, institute director, chair, and, most recently, Vice Chancellor for Health Affairs and Founding Dean. In each of these roles I have served as a mentor to junior faculty and have always had to "start from scratch" with each one. I am often astonished by the contradictory advice they have already received. Having also sat on institutional Promotion and Tenure committees, I have often been struck by the fact that junior faculty often can go several years in a new position before they have sought or been provided with any help toward promotion. It has always been my opinion that basic science departments in general perform this task better than clinical departments. In addition to advice on promotional issues, junior faculty members also need a great deal of general advice on such varied topics as time management and presentation preparation. This book by Drs. Geraci and Burton provides, for the first time, a very practical, common sense, and helpful approach to many aspects of professional success, and I believe it will be a valuable asset to all junior faculty members.

Academic success is not all about successful advancement. When you begin your first faculty position, you often are transitioning out of a residency or fellowship environment that is tightly organized and has clearly defined short-term goals (complete your rotations, finish your scholarly project, prepare for the boards, etc.). Training programs are required to have advising programs with mandated periodic feedback. With a faculty appointment, the path for success is often not as straightforward or clear. Drs. Geraci and Burton have developed several chapters that should be of great value to new faculty getting started, including a chapter dedicated to providing strategic advice for their first year on faculty.

Today there are very few "triple threats" left in academic medicine, so it is not surprising that most mentors are not equally competent in all aspects of the research, education, and service criteria for promotion. Without having provided recent service on an institutional promotion and tenure committee, mentors' perspectives on the topic are often dated. What was true for their careers is often not true for promotion today. Moreover, with the increasing size of departments and the increasing importance of clinical revenue to the academic enterprise, many chairs and deans no longer mentor junior faculty. As a result, most junior faculty members are now mentored by multiple individuals, each providing a specific aspect of advice. A junior faculty member's immediate supervisor is often a division chief, and that individual today is often under intense pressure for clinical productivity. These features of the current academic environment add greatly to the complexity of the process, and often present contradictory opinions to the mentee.

As outlined in the chapters of this book, advancement criteria in academic medicine and benchmarks for success have changed dramatically over the last few decades with a new appreciation for professional medical educators, the role of new teaching tools and information sources, as well as the need to adopt advancement yardsticks for the new generation of academic professionals with often different timetables, life style requirements, and family and personal commitments. New faculty members are often confronted with multiple demands on their time and little immediate advice on how to prioritize them. New promotion tracks have evolved, including a few academic clinician pathways that reward significant contributions in clinical practice and organization as well as quality and outcomes.

Perhaps the greatest change that has taken place during my professional career is the transition from a largely male-dominated profession to a junior faculty that today comprises an almost identical ratio of females to males. Unfortunately, however, the same is not true for faculty mentors, the large majority of whom are male. As a result, junior female faculty today often have more difficulty finding appropriate mentors for all aspects of their professional advancement. In addition they often face challenging dilemmas around balancing family and professional life. I was particularly pleased to find specific chapters in this book that address these critical issues.

This book is a much needed supplement to the mentoring process for junior faculty and their mentors. It provides many useful suggestions for addressing events likely to occur during the first few years of a faculty member's career. I would recommend that every medical school dean consider purchasing it for every new faculty recruit and that they consider it "required reading."

G. Richard Olds, M.D., M.A.C.P.
Vice Chancellor for Health Affairs and Founding Dean
School of Medicine
University of California, Riverside

Introduction

When Dr. Geraci first told me he planned to write a book to help guide young academic clinicians through the myriad and competing demands they face early in their careers, I knew it would be like nothing ever before written on the topic. He has proved me right.

During my more than six years of medical training, I have found no one more insightful, forthright, and generous with his or her wisdom—with more people at more career levels—than Dr. Geraci. As Chief of Medicine at the veterans hospital where I served as a chief resident, Dr. Geraci regularly met with young physicians at the start of their careers and helped them find a path to success and productivity that was beyond what any of them had ever envisioned possible for themselves. Those same physicians, including co-author Mary Jane Burton, M.D., would tell you they owe much of their success to the foundation of career-guiding principles provided to them by Dr. Geraci. Additionally, many of the trainees at the VA Medical Center and at the University of Mississippi Medical Center, where Dr. Geraci currently serves as Professor and Vice Chairman for Faculty Development in the Department of Internal Medicine, would tell you that no one has advocated for them with as much conviction, effort, and self-sacrifice.

I had the privilege of reading each of the monographs in this collection as it was being written. On so many of these occasions, I felt the book was being written specifically for me as I prepare to begin my faculty career. I imagine that, whether you are also just starting out or are well into your career as an academic clinician, you will feel the same way as you read each chapter. From what I have witnessed, as well as living with a father who has himself enjoyed a highly productive career as an academic clinician, the pressures seem only to become more intense as time passes. And as I met with and discussed my career issues, concerns, and challenges with Dr. Geraci, I often found myself saying (as so many of his trainees have said to him over the years): "I wish someone had told me these things before."

We all know that our responsibilities as academic clinicians involve—at a minimum—performing direct patient care, teaching trainees and students, producing scholarly work, serving on university and hospital committees, maintaining specialty certification, and complying with medical administrative duties. Additionally, each of us has responsibilities to fulfill to our family, friends, and community, as well as a responsibility to ourselves to maintain our own psychological and physical health. Each of these can, on their own, pose challenges, of course; but when considered *en masse*, they can seem daunting.

Moreover, for the junior academic clinician or one who aspires to meeting higher career goals, there are additional responsibilities: networking with colleagues, participating in specialty and subspecialty organizations, acquiring competency in making public presentations, developing writing skills, and demonstrating effective leadership at an institutional and, perhaps, local or national level. It should come as no surprise, then, that it is difficult (and sometimes seemingly impossible) for any academic clinician not only to maintain progress toward short- and long-term goals, but even to establish those goals in the first place.

Often, young physicians have a vague idea of the direction they would each like their career to take and a generic notion of how to get there. However, projects and additional responsibilities come along, while demands mount for more clinical productivity and administrative work; all too often these young physicians—each with a heart full of aspirations and the skill set to realize them—venture towards an area or an entire career where he or she is not fulfilled and does not excel. I have found myself and a number of my medical school classmates facing this very predicament during the past few years. A career as the local, regional, or even national expert in cardiac device placement, or genitourinary cancer, or interventional bronchoscopy might sound prestigious and lucrative when you don't have a guaranteed job after fellowship; but once you discover that your true joy is in another area entirely, such jobs can become virtual prisons where the promise of a fully engaged spirit is locked away, never to be realized.

The question, then, is how to avoid this outcome. How do we prevent the attrition of gifted, passionate academic clinicians to the armies of wasted potential? The answer is not a simple one, since each of our careers comes with a unique set of circumstances, but at a minimum it includes two elements: (1) a well-defined career plan; and (2) productivity toward the goals specified in that plan. Without the first, the young physician is subject to the whim of whichever competing demand is applying the most stress at the time. Without the second, nothing less than extraordinarily good luck will allow the academic clinician to achieve his or her objectives, regardless of how talented, brilliant, or charismatic that individual might be.

In *Notes for the Academic Clinician*, Dr. Geraci demonstrates, through a series of monographs based on three extremely productive decades as an academic clinician, what is entailed in developing a thoughtful, well-defined career plan—not one that merely identifies a few short- and long-term goals, but one that describes a thoughtfully crafted path that will most reliably and efficiently advance you toward those goals. Your journey begins with laying a solid foundation: identifying your values and preferences, and the things that you enjoy doing; crafting a vision of what you want your career ultimately to look like; recognizing what skills will be necessary and what will need to be accomplished in order to obtain those skills; and finding a mentor who is willing to invest time and effort in you. Once that foundation has been laid, building on it starts by choosing appropriate projects that progress you toward achieving your personal goals and ensuring that the efficacy of your efforts is maximized by effectively managing your time and keeping current with documentation. Mastering basic academic skills, including abstract writing, poster presentations, manuscript reviewing and medical writing are early steps needed to complete projects that will advance you toward achieving the goals you have set.

Such an overview makes avoiding the pitfalls of life as an academic clinician sound simple, but that is hardly the case. What makes the wisdom of this book so profound is that the author has personally experienced many of those unexpected bumps, turns and misdirections that occur, and has demonstrated the flexibility in his own career to adapt to them while maintaining productivity toward a set of ultimate goals. Subsequently, the knowledge learned from this experience has been conveyed to many young physicians, demonstrating measureable success of the concepts.

With training in internal medicine, hypertension, cardiovascular diseases, clinical and basic pharmacology, and critical care medicine, Dr. Geraci has served as a director of many courses and clinical rotations, associate residency program director, fellowship program director, clinical services director, chief of medicine, associate division chief for clinical operations and education, vice chair for faculty development, strategic plan consultant, and leader in national subspecialty committees and professional organizations. He has sat on numerous editorial boards and review committees for journals in cardiology, internal medicine, pharmacology, critical care medicine, and medical education. His extensive list of publications exhibits an impressive range: from basic to clinical science, from pharmacology to outpatient internal medicine and multiple medical subspecialties, from medical student education to master teacher reports. He has received awards and citations for his accomplishments as a clinician, a teacher, a researcher, and a supervisor/administrator.

Despite all these successes, what is most important to Dr. Geraci are the hundreds of physicians he has mentored and the many hundreds more he has advised at various points along their career paths. Dr. Mary Jane Burton, an infectious diseases physician and one of Dr. Geraci's mentees, complements the content of this collection by bringing her recent, in-depth experience to the monographs. As a clinical director, the first author on multiple peer-reviewed papers, and a mother of three small children, she has experienced the demands that many face, and is valued as a mentor herself among trainees and other young physicians at our institution.

The combined intent of Drs. Geraci and Burton in writing this book is to empower you to steer your career as an academic clinician in the direction you want it to take, rather than have it dictated to you by the competing demands on your time and energy. It's been my great pleasure to support their endeavor, and I am ever thankful to Dr. Geraci for his investment in producing a work that can now be available to academic clinicians everywhere. I know you, too, will be grateful. Read, re-read, and enjoy!

S. Calvin Thigpen, M.D.
Fellow, Division of Oncology and Hematology
University of Mississippi Medical Center

Chapter 1
Notes on Scholarship

Much of the collection that follows is related, either directly or indirectly, to increasing the career-long scholarly productivity of physicians who hold clinical or clinician-educator positions at a medical school or academic health center. As we began to assemble this collection, it occurred to me that I had neglected to clearly state the purpose of the book, or more specifically the importance of scholarship, for these critically important faculty members.

Several years ago, my then chairman of internal medicine asked me to give a noon conference to our residents about scholarship. My initial inclination was to then ask "What should I do with the remainder of the hour, perhaps explain the meaning of life?" After some thought, and abandoning the more pragmatic topics of how to make a poster or write an abstract (both important, but hardly sufficient), I aimed to focus the time with my younger colleagues toward conveying an understanding of both the definition, and importance, of scholarship.

I view scholarship as the unique product of scholars: those who study, learn, create, and convey information and understanding not available from other sources or individuals. The Boyer Model suggests scholarship includes four areas: (1) discovery (identification of new knowledge); (2) integration (translating new knowledge into forms that effect positive change in the general application of the discipline); (3) application (using the best knowledge, as produced and refined by scholars, in the practice of one's discipline); and (4) education (effectively conveying knowledge to others). I believe this to be the most useful available definition of scholarship for clinical faculty members, as it entails all that we do, and what we are asked to do, in the complex health care environments in which we work. Each of these areas has intrinsic value and is appreciated by most who seek to measure the scholarly productivity of physicians, though admittedly older thinking still undervalues many of the activities encompassed by this broad definition. Our medical residents had no difficulty accepting this definition, and in fact seemed comforted by its scope and inclusivity.

More challenging for me was to convey in this brief time frame why scholarship is so important. Again abandoning tradition (which has become my standard operating procedure), and again focusing on my favorite topic—the value of the individual, I thought about the times I had personally felt gratified by the various activities I identified as scholarship. The best strategy for my conference then became clear.

After gathering my young colleagues in a circle, I posed a short series of questions, related to their own career choices, for their consideration. First, I asked why they chose to become physicians instead of entering other fields that might be less costly, require less formal education and preparatory time, or provide an easier lifestyle or higher income. As expected, most hoped to commit their professional lives to improving the lots of others—whether for reasons of religion, philosophy, personal values, or a simple but sincere commitment to humanity. Next, I asked why they chose internal medicine as their specialty (and their specific subspecialties for those planning fellowship training). Although a few had difficulty getting past the more tangible aspects of an internist's life and practice, after some discussion most concluded that they believed they would be better internists than practitioners of other specialties; by being better at their work, they would make a greater contribution (scholarship of application). I then posed to them that if they could work in a more efficient setting—providing more of this benefit per unit of time or effort, would they choose to do so? A universal positive response was elicited. We then examined teaching—our institution is strongly committed to teaching as the very purpose of its existence—and asked why they saw teaching as such a valuable activity. Again some discussion ensued, but eventually we were able to agree as a group that each could extend the contribution they made by teaching their junior colleagues (scholarship of education). A few quickly saw the parallel and accepted the more global view that the real value of teaching was to *magnify their impact*; they saw that they could help one patient for one hour, or alternatively teach ten students during that hour, who might each help one patient each year for 30+ years of their careers, with that same effort.

These insightful residents made the rest of my task that day simple, for the remaining categories of scholarship (discovery and integration) had the same qualities as the ones they already acknowledged to be of value. By writing reviews and case reports, developing best practices, constructing career paths and contributing to evidence-based guidelines, the scholarship of integration magnified the impact of their efforts—more and better health care could be delivered as a result of this work than through direct health care delivery alone. By performing research, the scholarship of discovery magnified the impact of their work by delivering new knowledge to other scientists and practitioners, filling voids in our understanding of health and disease, or suggesting new ways to more efficiently and effectively improve the lots of patients, and people, everywhere.

I'd like to report having been blinded by all the light bulbs switching on as we reached the end of our hour together, but I was in fact quite gratified that the soft glow of a few exceeded my hopes when I first received this assignment from my chairman. A small step in the right direction, guided by these soft lights, is always better than wandering in the darkness.

————————◆————————

Scholarship is an impact multiplier. It allows each individual to make a greater contribution than he or she could otherwise make. As you read through this collection, I hope you will each keep in mind the simple truth of why we do what we do.

Chapter 2
Notes on Career Planning

In the continually changing world of health care in the U.S.—with more options, less time, more regulation, and less financial support—making the best career decisions for a young physician can be extremely difficult. Like most complex problems, having an organized approach, though not a guarantee of success, is the best strategy. Rather than answers, this chapter outlines the questions you need to ask, of yourself and others, to make sound career choices. The process is divided into four steps, though there can be overlap. Some steps can be addressed in parallel; others require a series approach to complete one step before moving on to the next. This is also a process you should repeat periodically, because situations change—as will you with time and experience. It is never too early to start a thoughtful, long-term approach to making the best career decisions—and never too late.

STEP 1: SELF-ASSESSMENT.

First, you need to understand where and who you are. You can't learn how to get from point A to point B without a candid understanding of where point A actually is. Through a rigorous self-assessment, ask yourself the following questions:

What am I good at?
Contrary to what your mother and third-grade teacher told you, you are not good at everything. None of us is. People in general are happier, and perform better, doing things they do well. It is OK to not be good at everything—it really is—but it is essential to know your strengths and limitations. For example, if three-dimensional thinking isn't your forte, imaging and certain types of medical procedures might not be your thing. If emergencies make you uncomfortable, concentrating on chronic disease management or prevention might be better than trauma surgery or critical care. If you

barely passed your math classes in college, a more humanistic, conceptual field might be better than a numerically intensive discipline such as nephrology. If you failed all your music lessons because your fingers wouldn't obey your brain, a cognitive field might suit you better than a procedure-intensive one. Be honest—you probably already know your strengths and weaknesses. Be willing to admit these things to yourself, accept them, and let this knowledge help guide your decision-making.

What do I like doing?
Get away from the standard, expected answers. We all like some parts of our jobs and dislike others. Think back, perhaps look at a calendar or pocket schedule, and try to remember the days you went home feeling great and the days you didn't. Examine those days—*why* were the good days good and the bad days bad? What part of those activities could be under your control, where you could choose to do more of the positives and fewer of the negatives? This is a distinct concept from days differentiated by whether your patients lived or died, whether you passed or failed an exam, or got a grant funded or rejected. Try to understand the *activities* that gave you pleasure, the *processes* that you enjoyed just because you engaged in them, whether or not the outcome was optimal each and every time.

Do you like teaching? Building clinical programs? Do you enjoy developing processes to make things run better? Organizing the disorganized? Meeting and interacting with people from other cities and schools? Do you enjoy the spotlight or prefer to be behind the scenes? Find yourself leading others, even when it's not in your job description? Does caring give you more satisfaction than curing? Do you find long-term relationships with patients more satisfying than the "high tech" side of medicine? Would you rather be in the bronchoscopy lab than the clinic? Do you see yourself wholly dedicated to treating the indigent, in a broad-based practice, or doing tummy tucks for celebrities who pay cash up front?

Most days we neither save a life, win a Nobel Prize, nor earn a million dollars. Routine activities are called routine for

5

a reason—they are what we do most often. Try to make choices that give you more of the good days and fewer of the bad ones, as *you* define them for yourself, based on this understanding.

Where does my job and career fit into my life?
Will your ultimate job selections be driven only by activities of the job itself, or are other factors (such as time flexibility, geography, income, or setting) very important to you? If you have children and want to read to them at bedtime each night, watch every soccer game and school play, don't be an intensive care cardiologist. If you feel just as content driving a Honda Civic as a Mercedes, and don't understand why someone who lives alone would want a 6,000 square foot house, perhaps income shouldn't be atop your priorities list. If your spouse wants to be within driving distance from his/her family, geography may be your starting place. Hate cold weather and think surfing is the only appropriate way to spend free time? Maybe Wisconsin shouldn't be a consideration. Do you work an 80-hour week even when you don't have to? If so, then you might think about positions where you would have broad responsibilities in different areas such as teaching, administration, and research in addition to patient care, where you will always have more to do.

It is very common to say "money doesn't matter"—and it doesn't, as long as you have enough. In fact, more than you need doesn't matter much. Whether driving a Subaru or Cadillac to work, you end up in the same parking space. But you need a car to get to work; a house in which you and your family feel comfortable; a rainy day fund; college tuition for the kids; and retirement savings. For some, additional financial rewards are important to create the lifestyle they and their families have always wanted, and that is an important consideration to acknowledge. Giving up other lifestyle values in pursuit of additional but nonessential income is generally a bad idea, but ignoring your real financial needs is a far worse one.

6

What do I value highly?
It may seem this question is repetitious, but in fact is the final one to address at this stage, since the others give you the raw material (knowledge) to answer it accurately. It is this value structure—highly personalized to every individual—that you should use to base present and future career decisions. Again, we all value good-quality patient care, think education is important, love our families, and want to make the world a better place, so such generic statements provide little insight. But if your good days involved running a successful resuscitation and bad days involved nine hours of clinic, there is a value judgment there. If you look forward to days where you teach in a classroom all morning, value is behind that feeling. If getting an article published, knowing that thousands of physicians will use what you wrote to help their patients, gives you particular satisfaction, you have made an important contribution according to your definition of value. Do you find you try to get patients with a particular problem into your practice because you feel their need for your work is great and you do an exceptional job in their care? You again will find personal values driving those actions.

We are very fortunate as physicians. Since there are so many needs that we *can* fill, we often have the luxury of selecting those we *choose to* fill based on our passions, preferences, and perceived rewards. We can make contributions in many different ways, and will do so more effectively when those contributions are ones we value the most.

Use the information you learn from answering these questions as your scale, to balance the positives and negatives of options that present themselves. There are no right or wrong answers to these questions, just truthful ones and...other ones.

STEP 2: CREATE A VISION.

When you are comfortable with your understanding of yourself and values (where you are now), the next step is to create a VISION of what you want, *and why you want it*. Is that vision consistent with your values? If successful, will you be doing the things you find rewarding, meeting your needs from your career, and making a contribution you deem important? Ask yourself the following questions:

What would be an ideal outcome for my professional life?
Do you see yourself as a highly respected physician within a community? A dean or chairman at a medical school? Maybe the person who developed the better mouse trap or designed an educational product that finally made acid-base understandable? Working in an office writing policy recommendations to guide medical care or resource allocation? Sifting through reams of data to clarify a best practice, based on evidence? Do you want to die with the longest CV, the largest bank account, the widest reputation, or the most patients thinking you were a great doctor?

It is crucially important at this stage to gather as much information as possible. What, exactly, does a pediatric neurosurgeon do all day? Do division chiefs get to spend their time doing the things you like doing? How much time does a medical director spend mired in situations you despise? Why would any physician ever want to be an administrator? How come department chairmen always look tired, depressed, and despondent? Is it reasonable to be grant funding-dependent in this day and age?

Though some information you discover will be objective (e.g., average tenure of a chairman of Internal Medicine in U.S. medical schools is about four years; average income ranges by specialty and geographic areas are published), most will be biased by personal opinion. You are assessing career satisfaction and, by definition, this is a subjective topic. Thus, the more opinions you hear the more likely you will be able to identify some truth you can use. Find people in those roles (or previously in those roles) and ask them what the job entails and what a typical day involves. What do they like, and dislike, about their jobs? Would they do it again or do they regret their choices? What, from their vantage point, is the future of this type of position—how has it changed over time, and how do they think it is likely to change by the

8

time you get there? What does it take to get there? What qualities, accomplishments, skills and abilities are needed—and important—for obtaining such a position (and succeeding in such a position, which often are two different issues)? What about job security, job availability, competition, and venue? You will find people very willing to talk with you, since everyone likes talking about themselves. Don't hesitate to ask the direct questions you need answered. Just remember you are asking people their opinions, and judge their statements accordingly.

Additionally, it is often best to make similar inquiries into alternative career choices. We rarely have the information we need when we must make such decisions; thus, when enough information is available, your second or third choice for a career might end up being the course you ultimately select to achieve the vision you have created for yourself.

Do I have what it will take to fulfill that vision?
You likely already know that everything comes with a price. Time, effort, personal sacrifice, risk, failure and recovery characterize every career path. Once you have an idea of what is needed, you must reconcile that vision with its price, and decide whether it is of sufficient value for you to pursue the path to that vision. Do you believe you have the abilities, resources, skills, patience, and commitment to achieve your vision? Having some doubts is normal, even wise, as no one can predict the future. However, once you determine that a given career goal will require success in your weaker areas, or spending considerable time and effort doing things you dislike and do not feel are valuable, you have hoisted red flags, suggesting you reconsider your vision and find out about other options before moving forward.

STEP 3: DEFINE YOUR ROUTE (MAKE A PLAN).

Once you have an idea of where you are and where you want to go, start planning the route. Rome really wasn't built in a day, and no one is likely to call you out of the clear blue sky and offer you an associate dean job just because you are a swell person. The "route" is really a series of interim

9

goals you will need to achieve, and each will require a certain amount of time, effort, training, and mentoring. Opportunity, of course, figures into all successful plans. Ask yourself the following questions:

What must I achieve to reach my goal?

In order to answer this question, you will need to get additional, specific information. Many of the requirements you identify will constitute necessary credentials ("getting your ticket punched") while some will also add to your tool set (skills and abilities), as discussed below. Review advertisements for the type of positions you seek, even if you are early in the process; though these certainly may change by the time you are a viable candidate for your ultimate career position, achieving competence or notoriety in many areas requires years, if not decades, of dedicated work.

If a predominately clinical practice setting is your goal, you may find that adding additional skills—procedural expertise, for example, or certifications in ancillary disciplines—will make you more competitive and provide more options for you. You might think about starting a product line or bringing a new clinical product to a hospital or practice, so some experience in these areas could bring worthwhile credentials. Involvement in local and state medical societies should also be considered. National professional organizations are increasingly producing CME and other products aimed specifically at the practitioner; their web sites and organizational publications can be very helpful toward identifying options and ways to obtain those skills.

If you are headed toward an academic career, learn the promotion and tenure policy for your school—and for other schools, which are often available on the web. Try to examine CVs of people who hold those positions, noting which credentials they have in common. From all these sources, specifically note peer-reviewed publications, research and grants, external acknowledgement (the "national reputation of expertise" factor), citizenship (intramural contributions related to committee work, projects, working groups and task forces), and educator goals. Get information from other schools, academic medical centers, research institutes, and government sources to see if another venue will be more conducive to your success.

If administration of some type is part of your vision, certificate or master's degree programs might be in order, or perhaps formal course work through professional societies. You will need to have a track record of both training and practical accomplishments/experience. And unless you were a business major in college, you probably have had little formal training in most relevant areas of administration.

If you hope to be a career-committed medical educator, courses and seminars on teaching, learning theory, and educational techniques and modalities will provide you with important skills and demonstrate your commitment. Negotiating a work schedule that has you teaching during much of your clinical time will help you gain a local reputation. Volunteering to give classroom sessions, even outside your primary department, will broaden that reputation. Look into both intramural and extramural training opportunities, and perhaps consider a certificate program or even an advanced degree (e.g., Master of Medical Education). Again, national professional organizations can be very useful resources to growing your skill set and enriching your reputation as a medical educator.

Research career development has been discussed by others and will not be repeated in this book, which focuses on clinical faculty development. Many publications and web-based resources can assist those wishing to structure a research career.

What new knowledge, abilities, and skills should I acquire?

Fortunately, we now live in an information age where opportunities for additional training abound. Both medical and non-medical options for training are easily discoverable. Many professional societies, your school's faculty development office, and programs at other medical schools made available to outside faculty, can provide much of what you will need to learn. The past ten years has seen an exponential growth in degree programs—M.P.H., M.M.E., M.B.A.—often specifically targeted at physicians that allow for distance learning and offer time-flexible programs. Remember, though credentials and history may get you a job, performance will keep you in the job. All employers have specific tasks they want completed by new hires—rarely are physicians hired for less directed purposes. You may have little time to acquire specialized skills after starting your new job, so mastering them in advance is always a wise approach.

Who is available, willing, and able to mentor me?
Of all the deficiencies in health care, the shortage of effective mentors may be the most profound, and most costly. In my opinion, lack of mentorship has led to more disappointments, failures, unrealized potentials and missed opportunities than has any other deficiency throughout recorded history. Mentoring is a challenging and time-consuming enterprise. There are few credentials (aside from an established track record) that identify good mentors, and no schools offer degrees in mentorship.

Everyone at every career stage can benefit from mentoring. Most of us should have more than one person in this role, each with different experiences and expertise. There are publications proposing how to choose a mentor, but these often focus on the career path chosen, with many articles and monographs available for researchers and relatively few for clinician educators, clinicians, and administrators. Generally, good mentors are more senior, with considerable professional knowledge and experience behind them and "connections" with people and organizations both within and outside your center; they have a personality with which you are comfortable discussing sensitive issues about yourself, your professional life, and sometimes your personal life as well; are willing and able to commit themselves to your success, and put some time and work behind that commitment; are people whom you trust to tell you the truth, whether or not the truth is pleasant; and whose integrity is worthy of your respect. Since mentoring is almost never financially compensated, mentors volunteer their time and work to their junior colleagues—a fact to keep in mind to assure your commitment to the relationship is at least as strong as theirs.

STEP 4: PAVE THE ROAD.

By this point, you should have a reasonable idea of what is needed for you to reach your goal. The final step, putting your plan into operation, involves specific activities that you can elect, negotiate, or agree to do, which fill these requirements and provide you with both the necessary capabilities and documentation. Again, such activities are highly specific to the path you choose, and a comprehensive listing is beyond the scope of this primer. However, there are some general principles applicable to most common plans:

Think in three-to-five-year increments. Develop reasonable interim goals, achievable and appropriate to each stage of your career.

Include major career and life events in your time line. For academics, time at rank and eligibility for promotion and tenure are important. Don't expect to get a 50-page paper written the month you will be delivering your second child. If moving to a new setting, allow six months (minimum) to get settled in your new home and learn your new job before starting on committees for the new cancer center. If you will be a program or course director, obtain the activities calendar up front and work your schedule to get your other duties done when the education activities (e.g., recruiting, orientation, accreditation site visits) are lightest. If coming out of training, your first year should center on transitioning your role—learning how to be an attending, or working in a non-teaching setting, or accomplishing the basic, day-to-day responsibilities as efficiently as possible; becoming efficient in your routine daily tasks "buys" you time to do the other things needed.

Determine which activities required by your present position will meet some of your development needs. If there are choices or options among your current position's required activities, select those that will contribute most to your career goals—the most "bang for the buck." If you are required to serve on one or more intramural committees, find out which ones might earn you credentials, or provide you additional experience and knowledge, in an area you have identified as important to meeting your goals. If you have a significant clinical load but plan a career in education, assess how much of that time you can spend in clinical teaching activities. If leadership is your goal, getting as broad an exposure to your local colleagues, other leaders, and recognition in all the practice and academic venues as you can is a solid approach.

Make an assessment of your flexible time. Assess not only how much flexible time you have (half day per week, a week per month, nights and weekends when not on call), but also how it is distributed (some time each month, month blocks, weekly, etc.). This should be re-assessed periodically, as it will be fluid (but most often decreasing) as you become more involved in your new role.

Proportion your time among the different activities identified in your roadmap. If you need to reach interim goals in multiple areas, it is often wise to have only one or two activities in each at a time. Some require time-intensive blocks but others will have peaks and valleys in their time requirements—a good plan takes these into account. Try to have some that are time-flexible, which you can work on an hour here or there, or the odd weekend, to use your time efficiently. Whenever possible, have several "irons in the fire" at once—you can never predict when an unforeseen road block will arise and, beyond your control, prevent progress on a given project. Have another activity on which you can concentrate to avoid wasting your precious discretionary time. Also, you will simply feel like doing some things at one time or another—take advantage of your psyche as much as possible: you will get more done when your interest is peaked toward a given task.

Set your own deadlines. Define them according to your schedule. If you have time now to work on a project not due for six months, do it now. If you are waiting for IRB approval before starting a study, maybe opt to take more on-call nights while you're waiting, to free up your schedule once the trial is approved. If you know you will be giving six lectures next academic year, block out library time, computer time, and practice time in increments to make best use of the year leading up to those lectures.

Leave yourself some uncommitted time. Try as much as possible to have some uncommitted time to seize unexpected opportunities that come your way. Almost no one does this. Most people look for opportunities only when they want them, and some of the best opportunities have brief windows of availability or come along very rarely. You may get an invitation to speak at a major meeting in six months, but your calendar is so full you don't see how you can come up with the hours needed to make your slides. Or you might get a chance to write for an evidence-based guideline because of a committee position you hold or from a colleague's recommendation who happens to know your interest and abilities. A society to which you belong may get an unanticipated committee or leadership opening. Opportunities missed are opportunities lost, so planning for the unexpected regarding your career can be as important as the other unexpected events for which you already prepare (with disability insurance, car insurance, etc.).

Make use of your mentors. Every interaction need not be a formal meeting. Get another opinion on whether you should accept or volunteer for a project. Tap into their understanding of how much value a given task will add to your resume, knowledge base, or professional contacts. Perhaps your mentor will know that an activity you believe will take much time and effort has really fairly trivial requirements, yet may open more doors for you in the future. Conversely, another opportunity that looks great on its surface may be laced with land mines, where your work will be great and the return modest. A quick email or phone call can save you from making errors of both omission and commission.

Plan, plan, plan. Electronic calendars are wonderful devices that will help you pull it all together and plan far into the future. Most professional meeting dates are set years in advance. The typical academic calendar covers an entire year. Some activities are reliably seasonal, while others are based on recurring time frames, such as grant submission deadlines and fiscal years. Forewarned is forearmed—try not to be surprised by finding April follows March next year, too.

Keep track of your accomplishments. Don't wait until you receive a notice that your annual performance evaluation is due in four weeks. Whether you choose to use your CV, a formal portfolio, or some other tool, add to it whenever you have something to add. Don't count on your memory. Have your mentors review this record periodically, both for organization and content.

Reassess frequently. Sometimes this is best done on your own; other times you should reassess with a mentor or supervisor. Every six months or so, spend an hour or two looking at your CV and your calendar. Perhaps keep a list of projects and goals and see which are working out and which are not. Most physicians spend more time analyzing their next new automobile purchase than their career progress. A little regularly scheduled maintenance can go a long way.

———————◆———————

As physicians, we typically seek dichotomous decisions: disease or normal, up or down, good or bad. Yet we all know that shades of gray are the rule, while black and white a rarity. Nothing can guarantee success anywhere in life, but success will be far more likely if you apply your intellect, organizational skills, and well-founded personal values to your career development.

Chapter 3
Notes on Writing a Career Development Plan

On every television news channel on the day of this writing, weather reporters are advising citizens to have a plan with which to deal with Hurricane Irene as it moves up the east coast of the U.S.: one that includes evacuation strategies, dealing with loss of electrical power and water, damage to property, and protecting vital documents and possessions. Two weeks earlier I had met with an advisor to review my insurance plan (disability, life, medical, long-term care, homeowners, automobile, liability, malpractice) to assure it would meet my family's current needs. On my calendar for the following week was a scheduled phone conversation with my family's financial planner, to adjust our investments as we weather the fiscal storm of the ongoing recession. The morning this draft was written, I logged onto a state medical site, having received an email reminding me to review my personal health maintenance plan. My niece and her husband had already started investing in a college savings plan for their first child, a one-month old daughter, Caroline. As our university hires more physicians from outside our area, each physician has a plan to find the best house, incorporating size, quality, location, safety, school systems, and taxes, for them and their families. And as I sat down to write this piece, I had just returned from running errands; a short trip that I planned out in advance in order to minimize both time and gasoline consumption.

All major, and many minor, activities and endeavors in our lives benefit from planning. Plans allow us to lower cost, avert disaster, maximize return, reduce mistakes, and achieve greater accomplishments than we could without a plan. Physicians are usually superb planners in some aspects of their lives, particularly their practices and day-to-day activities, as they seek to maximize the benefits given to their trainees and patients while minimizing the costs of time and effort. Most of us needed to plan carefully our scholastic and service paths to assure acceptance to medical school and its successful completion. So, clearly, we can develop and execute plans quite well.

Why then are so many academic clinicians without a thoughtful, comprehensive career plan? I have told hundreds of students, residents and fellows over the years that young physicians seem to spend significantly more time planning their next automobile purchase than they do their next career steps. I can only conclude that we—as senior colleagues and teachers—continue to fail you by neglecting to emphasize this critical need. Having not instilled the sense of its importance, the road to academic success has become littered with the career corpses of promising young physicians who failed to plan. We owe you our best attempt to correct this deficiency.

In Chapter 2, *Notes on Career Planning*, we describe a four-step process to understand our professional selves, define values, and set goals that are consistent with those values. In Chapter 6, *Notes on Choosing Projects*, we discuss an approach to make better choices about the activities to elect to undertake, and those to try to avoid, based upon a return-on-investment principle. Chapter 7, *Notes on Getting Started*, addresses several issues related to your first year on faculty. Other chapters in this collection address practical issues on specific activities and processes that should populate your career plan. Here, we address the structure of a well-developed career development plan that every young academician should create, and review and update at regular intervals.

Long-term goals are essential. You can never reach a destination if you don't know where that destination is. But the road to those destinations varies, with many possible wrong turns leading into dead ends; forks leading to long, sometimes unending routes to nowhere; and rocks and pot holes that can cause us all kinds of damage. Therefore, just as planning a long drive to a distant location would include milestones (intermediate points that confirm you are on the right road, and points where turns should be made), so too should your career plan include milestones, or intermediate goals, to assure you are on the route you have chosen.

Timeline for Career Goals

If you are just starting out, your ultimate career goals are likely to be 20 or more years in the future. With such a long journey, intermediate goals are critically important. First, they provide concrete, measurable achievements that you can use to define your progress. Second, they enable you to identify what you should be doing today, and tomorrow, and next month to move you toward your aspirations. Third, they help you assess opportunities down the line, to which you will be able to make longer-term commitments. Finally, they allow for periodic review and adjustment, as both you and the world in which you work changes.

A common approach is to define two-year, five-year, ten-year (perhaps), and long-term or ultimate goals in a formal career development plan. The shorter the time frame, the more specific and exact the goals should be. Two-year goals should reflect projects and activities you can work on now, can be completed with reasonable effort based upon your time availability, and be appropriate for someone at your present career stage. Five-year goals are usually a bit less precise: include goals that will require multiple steps or a longer commitment/greater effort to achieve; they should follow logically as intermediate steps between your two-year and longer-term goals. If you choose to include ten-year goals, these are most often obligate milestones toward your ultimate career aspirations—credentials, positions or experiences that are generally considered prerequisites for viable candidacy for that role or position. You may opt to define your time periods to coincide with your institution's time-at-rank schedule so that your goals focus more specifically upon academic promotion requirements.

Categories of Career Goals

How you categorize your goals is somewhat less important than your timeline, but still a useful feature of an effective career development plan. In general, using categories based upon traditional academic missions is reasonable. If your institution's promotion and tenure policy is organized by categories, then replicating that format in your personal career plan is the soundest approach (as among your goals is likely to be academic promotion). With the ongoing changes in academic health care, many will have jobs where less traditional categories, such as administration, information systems development, community service, or global initiatives, will be appropriate. At a minimum, the traditional academic health care missions of clinical care, education and research should be addressed, while others should be driven by your institutional requirements or career-specific aspirations.

If your goals are broad and your activities many, you may choose to incorporate subcategories to help keep the "big picture" in focus. Subcategories could divide activities into intramural and extramural, local and national or international (clinical), undergraduate and graduate (education), or business and clinical (administration). They are probably most helpful for your primary track/category, as you will likely have more projects and milestones here than in secondary areas.

Examples
Two-year goals should be very specific. Clinical examples of two-year goals include the number and types of review articles published; program development milestones (e.g., first patient in new center by January 1); committees you will join; extramural professional organizations you will join and the roles you will play initially in those organizations; guideline committees or national working groups you will join; journals for which you will review manuscripts; at which point you will reach what wRVU target; quality improvement programs in which you will participate. Education examples include what formal classroom teaching you will do for which programs; rotations and courses for which you will write a curriculum; extramural educational activities such as the Education Committee of a national society, NBME/USMLE or ABIM question writing committees; APDIM/ASP work groups; becoming associate program director. Research examples include establishing mentoring relationships with specific individuals; specific starter grants you will write and submit; clinical trials/protocols you plan to perform; what equipment, space, and resources you will obtain; courses on

grant writing and statistics you will take; initial research goals you will achieve. Administrative examples can include hospital-based committee work; courses you will take on finance or leadership; programs and centers you will direct and develop; and specific assignments you have accepted/will accept (chair of Medical Records Committee, director of the electronic health record implementation group, etc.).

Five-year goals should detail the expected progression of your two-year goals and include more complex and noteworthy achievements. Examples could include chairing a national guidelines committee; having published ten systematic review articles on clinical topics within your discipline; enrolling a target number of patients/year in your specialty center; obtaining training and added credentials in a new clinical area, procedure, or technique (including certification if available); establishing your subspecialty practice at an off-campus site; reaching an initial leadership position in a specific national professional organization; achieving competitive research funding in two consecutive cycles; becoming fellowship director; holding one or more journal editorial board positions; earning an MPH, MME or MBA degree; having a research line established with sequential studies that result in high-quality peer-reviewed publications; earning one or more teaching awards; becoming director of an undergraduate medical school course; establishing an expanded, defined referral network for your individual/specific practice.

Ten-year goals are generally those requirements you must satisfy to have a good chance of reaching your ultimate professional destination. These may not be needed for all career plans, but can be useful if you are reasonably certain that you want to work toward a very uncommon, ultimate academic role. These could include directing a profitable clinical center of excellence; chairing an NIH study section; becoming a residency or fellowship program director; or perhaps serving as a section or division chief. By this point in your career, you will have (hopefully) defined your primary career path, and ten-year goals should reflect that the majority of your time and effort will be dedicated to that goal. Secondary (lesser) efforts should be receiving less of your time, and those goals should be appropriately more modest.

Long-term goals constitute the eventual, "what I want to be when I grow up" compass reading, directing you to the "ultimate" career goals you are setting for yourself. These could be academic goals (program director, division chief, chairman or associate dean), clinical goals (direct a comprehensive disease management center; have a four-physician group in my subspecialty area as an independent service), educational goals (establish and direct a new primary care internal medicine residency; chair writing committees for the MKSAP), research goals (champion a functional clinical trials center in your discipline; obtain continuous NIH funding for your line of research, or have a functioning core lab for specific assays), and/or administrative goals (become Vice President for Medical Affairs, or Chief Medical Officer of an academic health center, Chairman of a department, or Dean). Although one long-term goal may be your primary interest, you should have long-term goals in more than one mission category (though probably more modest in subordinate categories), as few if any faculty physicians confine their activities to a single area.

Sample Templates for Career Development Plan
Normally I don't recommend templates for formulating things as individual as a personal career development plan. However, after multiple requests from our own faculty members, a few samples of how yours might look are included at the end of this chapter. Remember, however, that the best structure for *you* is the one that best organizes *your* professional activities, at the institution where *you* work, toward the goals *you* have set for yourself.

———————◆———————

Composing a thoughtful development plan, and reviewing and modifying it regularly, can be the single most important investment you make in your career, with unquestionably the highest return on your investment of any professional activity. Ask your mentors, supervisors, and other trusted individuals to help and advise you in this process.

SAMPLE TEMPLATE 1:

General Career Development Plan

	2-Year Goals	5-Year Goals	Long-term Goals
Clinical			
Intramural			
Extramural			
Education			
Intramural			
Extramural			
Research			
Intramural			
Extramural			
Administration			
Intramural			
Extramural			
(Other)			

SAMPLE TEMPLATE 2:

Career Development Plan Based on Specific Institutional Promotion Requirements

	2-Year Goals (Assistant Professor)	5- to 6-Year Goals (Associate Professor)	12-Year Goals (Professor)	Long-term Goals
Category 1				
Group A activities				
Group B activities				
Group C activities				
Category 2				
Group A activities				
Group B activities				
Group C activities				
Category 3				
Group A activities				
Group B activities				
Group C activities				
Category 4				
Group A activities				
Group B activities				
Group C activities				

SAMPLE TEMPLATE 3:

Clinician Educator Career Development Plan

	2-Year Goals	5-Year Goals	10-Year Goals	Long-term Goals
Clinical				
Hospital/Inpatient				
Office/Outpatient				
Education				
Students				
Residents/Fellows				
National				
Research				
Education Research				
Multicenter Trials				
Administration				
Hospital				
University				

SAMPLE TEMPLATE 4:

Clinician Investigator Career Development Plan

	2-Year Goals	5-Year Goals	Long-term Goals
Clinical			
wRVU goals			
Education			
Teaching			
Research			
Multicenter Trials			
Collaborations			
Intramural Grants			
Extramural Grants			
Administration			
Research Administration			
Other			

Chapter 4
Notes on Leadership

I was asked by some of my colleagues to include a discussion on leadership in this collection. I believe some of the requests were with the hope that a monograph could help them learn to become leaders. Others, I believe, wished to learn how to identify an effective leader. I do not think either of these are achievable goals in a simple essay. Perhaps the best use of this chapter is to help individuals identify whether they are natural leaders by providing a summary of the qualities, attitudes, and skills that lie at the core of effective leadership. A self-evaluation, based on this guide, is recommended before embarking on the long and challenging road towards traditional leadership positions.

I do not believe leaders can be created. Leaders are born and raised, grow to become people of character, and inherently experience deep personal satisfaction from helping others achieve success through a very special service to them. "Leadership education" does not, in my opinion, impart the essence of effective leadership, but rather teaches skills and techniques that leaders can use to carry out their work more effectively. Some actually teach management, which is clearly distinct from leadership; management should never be confused with true leadership.

There are as many concepts of leadership as there are people who have pondered the topic. The military has sought to develop leaders since the inception of formal military education and training programs. The business and financial worlds have made leadership development into…a business, in and of itself. Politicians claim leadership abilities almost daily, but usually cite successes in other roles as supporting evidence. Books, courses, workshops, consulting companies, professional organizations, colleges and universities all claim to train leaders: one could easily spend half of his or her time "learning" to become a leader. I have been a student of leadership all my life, as I believe most of the solvable but unresolved problems in human society originate from a lack of effective leadership. I have had rich opportunities to study leadership in health care (and particularly academic health care) at the eleven U.S. medical schools and host of academic medical centers where I trained or worked during the past 35 years, having observed some effective leaders and many more ineffective so-called leaders. Whenever the opportunity presented, I have read books, attending lectures and courses, and discussed the topic of leadership with deans, chairmen, division directors, CEOs, VPMAs, and health care administrators, seeking to understand leaders and leadership.

A Model of Leadership: Character, Vision, Competence

From all these experiences, component qualities of the effective leader have coalesced into a model (a theory, really) that I have tested against events and individuals to determine if the model holds true; whether violating the principles of the model resulted in adverse outcomes; and whether upholding the principles led to demonstrable benefit—during both routine and unusually trying situations. The following is a "tripartite model" of leadership (my apologies to Aristotle) that you should consider if you think leadership may be in your future.

Character. Leadership begins with character: integrity, honesty, humility, respectfulness, justice and fairness, and commitment to those who are led and to shared values and causes. There is no substitute for character, and it is not something you can learn or acquire. Integrity, as defined here, refers to consistency of thought and behavior, regardless of circumstances. I think of this as doing the right thing under all circumstances, whether easy or difficult, enjoyable or painful, popular or damning, and whether or not anyone else ever knows what you have done. Integrity cannot be compromised, because when compromised, it ceases to exist.

Honesty is a sine qua non—nothing will erode a leader's credibility faster than getting caught in a lie. Honesty is not just truthfulness of words, but also of spirit and intent—a

29

quality that we commonly identify as sincerity, but which is in fact honesty of mind and action.

Humility is an underappreciated quality (while hubris is the ultimate sin of a leader). It allows you to learn, to weigh facts objectively, and to never judge based on your own feelings, opinions, or inflated self-impression when these conflict with the evidence.

Respectfulness defines the values that underlie all inter-actions leaders have with those who are led as well as with others. A true leader can be effective if he or she genuinely respects people for their intrinsic human value and, more specifically, the people he or she is leading for the value they bring to the group or organization. Respectfulness can-not vary based on whether the leader likes or dislikes the individuals being led. Narcissism, unfortunately, is far more common among those holding leadership positions, and since narcissism by its very definition undermines respect-fulness for others, it is often a defining characteristic of failed leaders.

Justice and fairness grow from respectfulness, as a nat-ural product of inherently valuing the people you lead: A common mistake here is to confuse justice with kind intent: many new leaders seek to earn the favor of their followers by using their position to impart gifts of one type or another. True leaders, particularly in academic medicine, have little if any of their own "capital" to spend as they choose, but are stewards of the group's capital, which requires them to con-sider total group benefit when expending those resources.

Commitment to those who are led and to the shared val-ues and goals of the group is manifested most often through self-sacrifice: subjugating one's own personal and career needs in deference to the needs of one's followers. This is fundamental and all too often absent from "popular leaders." Personal courage, usually manifested in putting one's self at risk for the benefit of the followers, is the quality that, in part, allows for the behavior of self-sacrifice. The success of the group (as opposed to the success of the leader) must be paramount. *Leadership is service to those led.*

Vision. "Vision," of course, is a component of most leadership models. Being able to see where the group or organization needs to go and identifying the best route to get there distinguishes the true leader from the effective manager. But true leadership vision encompasses much more: it includes the ability to see the truth, to peer through the haze of politics, emotions, and personal concerns, and thus visualize the actual facts, issues, challenges, and opportunities that exist. A leader must be able to accurately discern issues influencing process decisions for the group, and the true qualities of each group member—to be able to see whom someone really is, and understand him or her to the degree needed to lead each individual effectively. Finally, a leader needs to be able to "see" ahead—to understand the path sufficiently in order to anticipate hazards, prepare for possible obstacles, and identify alternative routes to reach the destination.

Competence. This quality describes the ability of a leader to solve problems, effect compromise, empower and delegate responsibility with authority, protect from outside attacks, and assure the group members' time and effort are never wasted but instead are maximized to produce the greatest good for the least effort. Competence will always include extensive knowledge of the field, environment, institution and people that could affect the activities and outcomes of the group. Exercising competence is the tactical skill that most observers witness, and is often the major determinant of a positive opinion of someone's leadership abilities. It is true that most interactions leaders have with their followers tap into this ability: a need for the leader to solve problems the individuals cannot solve themselves. Of course, the details of the specific skills needed will vary with the environment, type of school or medical center, leadership level (e.g., division chief vs. dean), and other factors. Of the three components, competence is the one area where training and experience can lead to skill enhancement.

———————◆———————

Arguments can certainly be made that many effective leaders have other qualities and skills that may enhance their abilities in one or more areas, or contribute to the "gravitas" some feel leaders should exude. I believe, however, that if one religiously demonstrates the highest character, possesses clear vision, and continually strives for competence in the day-to-day operations of the group or organization, everything else will follow naturally and with little deliberate effort.

If you are considering leadership positions in your future academic career, spend a few moments asking if the above description applies to you. If so, and if you are willing to make the sacrifice, there is truly no more satisfying an experience than to lead talented young physicians, students and staff toward success. If not, do not be discouraged; academic medicine presents many career options that contribute greatly to the well-being of others, and these alternate roles are no less important than traditional leadership positions. You will be happier, and make greater overall contributions, in a role that fits with your abilities, personality, and values.

Chapter 5
Notes on Finding a Mentor

Finding a mentor is easier than finding a spouse—but not significantly so. There have been many attempts to define effective mentoring, identify tools that can improve the mentoring process, or describe details of mentoring relationships commonly identified as successful. Most publications on physician mentoring relate primarily to those developing laboratory science careers, but mentoring is essential regardless of your career path. All mentoring relationships involve trust, commitment, and respect; beyond these similarities, however, there are as many different relationships as there are people who enter into them.

Most academic physicians who have both been mentored effectively and returned that service as effective mentors generally agree on a number of points you may find helpful:

First and foremost, try to accurately define your mentoring needs. Most young academic physicians need one or more individuals to advise them on general career decisions, including selecting projects and academic activities, assuring progress toward promotion and tenure, and allocating their time and energies most effectively. A career mentor should be able to understand your long-term professional goals, and how your work responsibilities interface with your family and personal life. Initially many will find a clinical mentor of significant value—a physician seasoned and experienced in your field with whom you can discuss challenging cases or receive guidance on procedures or specific techniques. Anyone starting a clinical or bench research career needs mentoring in general aspects of investigation (study design, formulating hypotheses, statistical testing of data, etc.), specific techniques to be used in the laboratory or clinic (as well as securing collaborators and obtaining access to shared equipment and resources, physical plant space, and support personnel), maneuvering through the convoluted paths of regulatory approval, and identifying and successfully competing for funding. A mentor for educators can be particularly helpful, not only to help you refine your teaching skills, but in developing courses, curricula, and programs that meet current educational standards. Having a mentor who can facilitate your entry into the national/international arena through networking at meetings, seminars and extramural professional organizations can also be extremely valuable. There may be considerations in your personal life that figure heavily into professional issues—such as a special needs child or caring for an infirmed parent, for example; an advisor with similar experiences can be of great assistance as you try to meet all the demands on your time. Some of you will need encouragement while others may need a dose of reality from time to time. Thoughtful introspection is the first step—figure out what you need *first*.

Understand that one person will not fill all your mentoring needs. Senior faculty will have different skill sets, knowledge and expertise that can be helpful to you in one or more areas. However, particularly when embarking on an academic career where you may work in clinical, educational, research, and administrative roles, most new academicians will need a number of mentors to address all their needs for advice and counsel. Some institutions employ formal mentoring committees to operationalize this model, while others may encourage (or initially assign) a "primary" mentor/advisor who helps you identify others to meet your specific needs. Develop relationships with a number of experienced faculty members at your institution and perhaps with some at other schools or medical centers, whether or not you enter into formal mentoring relationships with all of them.

Your mentoring needs will change over time. As your career develops and you venture into new professional areas or become more sophisticated and specialized in one or more areas, expect to identify new mentoring needs that will require different/additional advisors to counsel you. This is the rule rather than exception, and whether based on a new line of research, a growing role in leadership, or changing responsibilities toward new clinical activities, expect to need additional mentors as your career develops.

There are no mentoring credentials that matter except a track record of successful mentees. Never assume that the best mentors are the most published, or most highly funded, or politically most advanced members of the faculty. They may be, but these achievements do not equate to being an effective mentor. If possible, speak with colleagues more knowledgeable than yourself about senior faculty members' reputations, to help identify those with whom other junior academicians have had success—particularly in the areas where you have identified personal needs. Talk with those mentees, and ask questions that you feel are particularly important for your development. Are they available? Approachable? Can they be counted upon when needed? How did they help with their mentees' successes (and perhaps more importantly with their failures)? Were confidences kept? Did they keep their word? Was their advice sound, and perhaps supported by other individuals? Obviously, every mentor has a first experience—eliminating the possibility of a demonstrable track record. But most people never know whether they will be effective mentors until they try— and you'd rather not be the one who helps them discover that mentoring isn't for them!

Learn about potential mentors in advance of your first contact. Review their CVs, search the published literature, use web search engines to find out about their professional and perhaps other (e.g., philanthropic, community) activities. Speak with their contemporaries, their students and trainees, and others who have known and worked closely with them—and perhaps those who chose not to work with them. Try to ascertain how a potential mentor is likely to deal with the types of issues you anticipate facing in your early career. Is he someone who will advocate for you with your division chief or chairman? Does she regularly access extramural professional contacts for her mentees? Has his career track been similar to the one you seek? Is her personality a good match to yours? Is he generally on campus, or constantly traveling to professional meetings and seminars? And most importantly, were previous mentees successful under her tutelage?

Establishing and Defining a Mentoring Relationship
As you begin exploring potential mentors, ask to meet with him or her to discuss a possible mentoring relationship, and set an interview time when you can both fully devote yourselves to the conversation. Most people will be receptive to an initial discussion, often even if they don't know you that well. Being asked to mentor is an honor, though not one that can universally be accepted. It's a good idea to provide your CV in advance, so he or she can begin to put together an understanding of who you are and what you have done professionally. Have your thoughts organized before your first meeting—be able to describe your career plans, aspirations, self-perceived strengths and abilities, and honestly identified shortfalls that you are trying to correct. Be prepared to answer questions—some of which may seem personal, but which may give your identified mentor more understanding of your values and how your career fits in with other aspects of your life.

If this initial meeting goes well, send your potential mentor a thank-you note or email, and *ask for a follow-up meeting to discuss specifics of your future interactions.* Ask about time and availability; how frequently you should have regularly scheduled meetings; what types of issues/areas he or she feels qualified to provide advice; what types of resources he or she can provide for you or assist you in obtaining for yourself; and what his or her expectations will be of you. Discuss philosophy of credit on joint projects (authorship, investigator status), as this varies greatly among institutions and individuals. Also explore how long a commitment you are both prepared to make initially, and perhaps agree on a time when you will jointly re-examine the mentoring relationship and decide on its future. In essence, you are formulating and entering into a contract with your mentor, and the more detail and clarity in that understanding, the more likely your relationship will be productive and mutually fulfilling.

36

Realistic Expectations, Responsibility, and Etiquette

Once you have established a mentoring relationship, commit to making it successful by adhering to the following principles:

Live up to your end of the bargain. Your mentors are largely donating their time and effort to help *you* successfully reach *your* professional goals. Some of course will gain professionally from your relationship with them, through expanded research activities and publications, but for the most part the hours of time contributed by a devoted mentor typically receive little formal acknowledgement. Therefore, it is absolutely essential that you do whatever is necessary to fulfill your commitments, whether it's meeting milestones for project completion, attending meetings on time, performing agreed-to training and literature research, or fully preparing in advance for your conferences with your mentor.

Always be respectful of your mentor's time. Remember that, for the most part, mentoring is an uncompensated activity, and the most sought-after mentors tend to be some of the busiest people on campus. Try to limit email length. Don't leave things to the last minute, nor expect responses to your emails the same day. When you need your mentor's input on an *ad hoc* basis, try to compile all your relevant questions, express them succinctly, and perhaps have the options you are considering written out in advance.

Keep the relationship professional. Many people develop caring relationships with their mentors, and these can be very rewarding experiences. But a mentor isn't your parent, buddy or girlfriend. Certainly express your gratitude for his or her time and efforts, but giving personal gifts, getting involved in their personal lives (beyond discussions necessary for your professional decisions), or other activities implying more than a mentor-mentee relationship is not only inappropriate, but can be frankly destructive on multiple levels.

Be independent and accountable. *You* must do most of the work to develop *your* career. Your mentor can assist, advise, and make very important contributions to your progress; it is *your* responsibility, however, to complete the tasks, projects, and work to earn your way to where you want to go. He or she can advise you on issues germane to a decision you need to make, but ultimately it is always *your* decision to make. Your mentor may be disappointed if you fail—but you will be the one living with the consequences of your failures. Your mentor is the *second* most important person in this relationship.

Keep in mind these caveats to mentor/mentee relationships. Remember, mentors are people too, with their own biases and interests. Your independence includes an acknowledgement of this fact. With any advice you receive from your mentors, always consider that they do often glean tangible benefits from your work, including authorship and work you perform in their lab, office or discipline. Before embarking on projects or other additional commitments of time and effort, critique their advice based upon your overall career plans, and be confident that whatever you are advised to do will bring you closer to your professional goals.

————————◆————————

Academic physicians who have participated in long-term mentoring relationships almost always see them as the most rewarding, valuable experiences of their careers. Those who received high-quality mentoring from a thoughtful, committed, sincere senior colleague usually become the best mentors of their generation. Learn from the experience. Pay attention not only to the substance of the advice and support you receive, but also the process—the art of good mentoring. Before you know it, your junior colleagues will be asking you to mentor them, and you will have the honor and privilege of "paying it forward."

Chapter 6
Notes on Choosing Projects

In almost every situation requiring a decision, we make value judgments—assessing, as best we can, the cost (be it money, time, effort, political capital, or whatever) and benefit (income, notoriety, good will, benefit to society, professional advancement, etc.), and determine which of the available options is the best value: the greatest benefit for the lowest cost. We do this for small things, such as deciding which route to drive to work, and large things, such as buying a house or ranking residency programs. This same basic concept of value, or stated more operationally, return-on-investment, is also applicable to decisions related to your academic career.

You will have many different types of opportunities for projects and activities throughout your professional life. These will be as diverse as being asked to give a lecture to students or residents on a specific topic, joining a committee or task force, collaborating on a writing project such as an expert consensus statement, or participating in a multi-center collaborative research study. With some of these opportunities you will have little choice but to accept, as they will be assigned or "strongly recommended" by your division director or department chair. For others, you may have a choice from a group of options (such as selecting three lecture topics off a curricular list for a fellowship program, or volunteering for one work group out of several needing new members). A last group of activities is totally elective, where you may be invited to participate in a task force by a national professional organization, or hear about a campus work group looking for volunteers to make curriculum recommendations or contribute to the strategic plan for your department; some you may need to specifically seek out, e.g., by asking a senior colleague to recommend you to the NBME for participation on a question-writing panel, or contacting the president of a professional organization to volunteer for a specific committee. Each of these opportunities needs to be evaluated in terms of its return-on-investment.

COST

The first required assessment is cost. What will you need to do—how much time, effort, disruption to your present schedule, travel, potential lost income or consumption of time from other activities—to fulfill the requirements for this project? This is not always easy to determine. A committee might only meet once each quarter, but the work project could consume many hours out of committee for activities such as policy development, fact-finding, literature research or draft writing. Conversely, you may need to write only a few paragraphs on a topic with which you are very familiar to be a contributing author on a consensus statement from a major professional organization in your field. Some activities, such as IRB membership, have ongoing, heavy time requirements and should be considered only under specific circumstances and for a limited appointment period; others might just need basic recommendations from a physician in your specialty and take only an hour here and there over the course of a year. Key features to consider in assessing cost include:

- **Timeline** (whether you will have the time in the proscribed period to complete a given task, given your routine duties and assignments such as service months and prescheduled classroom teaching);
- **Time flexibility** (i.e., is it work you can mostly do according to your own schedule, or will you have many scheduled meetings and other activities around which you must work your other activities, or travel out of state), and timing of scheduled duties (e.g., weekly Monday meetings in the middle of your major RVU-generating clinic);
- **Other simultaneous activities** related to your academic productivity (e.g., whether you already have similar projects in process and therefore need to secure additional resources to undertake another);
- **Predictability** of project requirements (more is better);
- **Co-workers** with whom you will be working (which could make things either easier or more difficult);

- **Your previous experience** with similar types of projects (we all get better and more efficient with experience);
- **Supporting resources** available either from the project sponsor or locally (e.g., librarian, data, support personnel, perhaps special software or IT support);
- **Lost income** has become a real issue when your salary is RVU-based. Activities that will necessitate cancelling a significant number of clinics or study reading days should be considered in your cost analysis;
- **Political costs** are less objective and often harder to quantify. Committing to one project (or choosing not to commit) could be taken by some as negative—a trusted advisor, immediate supervisor, or close colleague could view your choice negatively for a host of reasons;
- **Other costs** specific to the activity you are considering.

If this is a new type of activity for you, advice from senior faculty and mentors can be critically important. Try to find someone who has performed similar projects, and the more similar their experiences to the one you are considering, the better. Knowing, for instance, that a given journal asks for three or four reviews each month is a vastly different expectation for an editorial board member than one which asks for only three or four reviews each year. Finding out that the committee you are considering is chaired by someone who talks incessantly, has poor leadership skills, is disorganized, and basically wants the committee members to do the work while he or she takes the credit, is key information on cost (and benefit). You may also need to specifically ask about support from the sponsoring organization—regarding literature search and article acquisition, literary editing, etc. for a group writing project, or administrative support to set up conference calls and record meeting minutes for a leadership role in a professional organization.

It is rarely possible to make a complete and accurate assessment of total cost of a given activity or project, but the more you know the better your chance of making a good decision.

BENEFIT

The second part of the equation is benefit—the return on your investment. As difficult as it can be to determine cost, potential benefit assessment can be even more challenging. It helps to look at categories of benefits as different types of projects, undertaken at different career stages, may have very different benefits for you.

- **Direct credit** is the most obvious benefit you will receive for completing the project—where it will fit on your CV, or what promotion criterion it will satisfy. Activities directly related to your faculty track requirements, particularly when you have few or no projects in that category, is an obvious valuable benefit.
- **Multiple category activities** fulfill more than one promotion requirement. Serving on the education committee of a major national organization, for example, may "count" toward your achievements in education, service, and national reputation categories.
- **Downstream projects** comprise another potential benefit. Often, the body of work you do for a given activity can be used for additional projects at a later time. For instance, writing a section for an evidence-based guideline, published by a major international professional organization, is a prestigious clinical activity that will clearly identify you as an expert in your field. It will also consume a huge amount of your discretionary time for weeks or months—a high cost. However, the knowledge you gain from your literature research could be the basis for a number of new lectures and workshops you could present. Smaller but important articles, where you expand from your writing on the guideline, could add a number of publications to your CV. With publication of the guideline, you may be asked to give national presentations—both about the guideline itself, the general topic, or perhaps a particularly unusual section of your work that has research potential or novel applications to another specialty or another disease-specific interest group. You might even develop a new research area,

addressing questions you would never have considered before your guideline work. So, although the two hundred-plus hours you spend on researching and writing your section of a guideline might initially seem to be an unacceptably high cost, the return is often well worth the effort, if you fully exploit the opportunity.

- **Institutional benefit** applies to some projects or activities that are very important to your medical school, department, or hospital; completing them could open doors for you within your institution. Success can lead to opportunities, though long-term benefits can be hard to predict. Internal projects can have hidden and unsuspected responsibilities, so the cost may not be predictable. Conversely, service (previously referred to as "citizenship") is an expectation of most faculty members, and some contribution beyond your practice and teaching is likely part of everyone's responsibility.

- **Networking benefits** of certain activities are often under-appreciated. Everything you do with experts and physicians outside your home institution introduces the potential benefits of extramural networking. Those who chair committees and writing groups, direct work groups preparing exam questions or best practice documents, and edit journals are always looking for reliable, competent, creative people willing to volunteer their time and effort toward a project they value. Unfortunately, too many volunteers fail to submit timely reports or meet the mandate of their charge; others over-commit, or discover the work is far more demanding than they expected, and fall short of expectations. Young people who perform admirably on an important project are remembered by those responsible for that project—and those selected to run one major project are usually asked to run others. When asked to put together a group for their next endeavor, they may remember you and your earlier work— resulting in an opportunity you would not have otherwise been offered.

- **Reputation** is something you will be building throughout your career. Ever wonder how the famous people in your field became famous? Certainly, many have performed ground-breaking research that earned them notoriety. However, others have seized opportunities, performed well, been noticed by those in leadership, and worked their way up the ladder to more influential positions at their home institution or within organizations. An important project, such as an evidence-based guideline or article series on a timely topic, could make you a sought-after expert in a surprisingly short time.

- **Financial benefits** are fairly obvious. Some work you get paid for, some you don't. Except as proscribed by your particular compensation plan, intramural activities almost never pay you for additional work, though projects that grow your practice can have obvious financial rewards. Some extramural projects, particularly if they contribute to a revenue-generating product of a professional organization, may provide an honorarium; these however are usually modest and rarely compensate you for your work at a competitive rate. Compensation for industry work (speakers' bureau, consulting, etc.) pay better, but growing concerns about conflict of interest and professional ethics are rapidly making such relationships less attractive. Indirect financial benefit, such as fully reimbursed travel expenses, may be of value if you combine your work trip with other personal activities, but again these are modest at best and are increasingly considered as financial compensation that you must report in Conflict of Interest disclosures. Overall, few of the commonly-available professional activities are likely to provide significant direct financial benefit.
- **Personal fulfillment** is uncommonly discussed, but an important consideration. Some projects are fun to do, or personally gratifying in other ways. This is an individually-defined benefit, and hard to quantify when trying to make a return-on-investment assessment. Yet these activities may be the most fulfilling you choose to undertake. Don't neglect this benefit in making your decisions.
- **Titles** make some roles look appealing, but beware. There is an old saying in business: "A title is what they give you to get you to work for free." Although this is not universally true, be wary of titles early in your career.

Most young academicians are enticed by holding a "Director," "Associate Director," "Committee Chair," "Supervisor," or other ego-enhancing title. Most titled positions, whether hospital-based, practice-based or medical school-based, require a significant amount of administrative responsibility and work. Unfortunately, some institutions survive on a steady diet of young faculty members, burdening them with administrative functions that consume their discretionary time and prevent their essential early development for future research and scholarship success. There are only two situations where a titled position will be of benefit to you at the beginning of your academic career: first, if your primary career plans focus on medical administration (e.g., chief of staff, chief medical officer, vice president for medical affairs); and second, if your career plans specifically include moving up along that particular pathway (e.g., a goal of becoming an associate dean via a vice chair for education and residency program director position, starting with an associate program director position). Otherwise, it is best to avoid such positions if at all possible until other aspects of your career scholarship are well developed—usually three to five years after joining the faculty.

Some activities can have multiple benefits, but there is no common denominator that allows you to make precise judgments. Weigh the above factors, and others you may identify, in estimating how much return you can expect on your investment.

OTHER CONSIDERATIONS

A few other factors should be considered in selecting projects. One is **opportunity**. Great projects rarely come around when you are looking for them. Some may only come along once in a decade or in a professional lifetime. Invitations to participate in high profile, national or international expert groups are an example, particularly early in your career. Others include leadership openings in professional organizations, invitations to become an investigator with an elite group of scientists in your field (say, as another site in a multicenter study), or initial involvement with an organization such as the national board of your medical specialty. You will always be busy, and able to list a dozen reasons to refuse such opportunities. But opportunities missed are opportunities lost; figure out how to make it work so you can accept invitations that will provide exposure that you might otherwise never realize.

Another factor is **novelty**. Even though you may have a pretty good idea where your career is going, you may have other areas of interest that can be worth investigating. Health care, medical science, policy, and politics are constantly changing. An unusual opportunity can sometimes enlighten you about possibilities you've never before considered, and suggest a development path that could be better for you than your existing one. Keep an open mind.

————————◆————————

There is no fail-safe mechanism for selecting professional projects. But a systematic, considered approach, thoroughly examining costs and benefits, will serve you best throughout your career.

Chapter 7
Notes on Getting Started
(*Your First Year on Faculty*)

Your first faculty year is easier than your intern year or your first fellowship year, but only marginally so. Starting a new role, particularly at a new institution, has many of the same issues you faced during other "first" years in your career. However, as opposed to medical school or training programs that have fairly objective criteria for success and involve a finite time commitment, your first faculty year has greater long-term implications arising from more subjective evaluations of you and your work. You no longer have the "protection" of being a trainee in an approved program; no work-hour limits; few if any superiors officially concerned about your mental or physical health; and you are now subject to the expectations of more than one individual (e.g., chairman, division chief, hospital CEO, practice manager, and others). You are now an employee, and despite all the talk about the value of professional growth, importance of higher scholarly aspirations, and individual best intentions, as an employee your institution—working through your superiors—will want as much from you per salary dollar paid as possible. We work in a capitalist system, after all, with constantly shrinking resources available to support ever increasing workloads.

Your first three-to-four years on faculty will define the rest of your career. After that, your practice is established, your role within your institution will be defined, and people's impressions of you will be set in their psyche. If you had a "start-up package" or salary guarantee period, both have most likely ended by three years (or sooner) at most medical schools and academic health centers. If you have not started your research and obtained or made significant progress toward securing external funding, established yourself as a high-quality educator, shown leadership potential, or succeeded at the initial phases of publishing and national involvement, you are very unlikely to have the discretionary time or inclination to do so after this period. Moving to a new institution might provide a second chance, but remember starting over comes with its own price, and is an option that will require considerable thought, examination, time and effort on your part. More extreme steps (such as returning for additional residency or fellowship training) may be your only other option if your early years fail.

Prior to starting your first job as a faculty member, you should formulate your own career development plan and insist on as much detail in your contract/agreement letter as possible.

Career Development Plan

Think through and formulate a *detailed* career development plan (see Chapter 3, *Notes on Writing a Career Development Plan*). You can never be sure you are headed in the right direction if you don't know where you are going. Hopefully, you constructed such a plan before negotiating your contract but, if not, do so as soon as possible. This is your roadmap to guide decisions on individual projects and duties that you will be offered or asked to do. Many, many promising, talented, enthusiastic young academic physicians have terminally derailed their careers by losing control early, overcommitting their time and energies in directions that contribute little to their professional development, to realize only too late that the expected benevolence of their immediate superiors was subjugated by the more immediate needs of covering services, bringing in clinical dollars, and satisfying their superiors within the administrative hierarchy.

Contract Stipulations

Just as in litigation, "If it isn't in writing it didn't happen," so insist on as much detail in your contract or agreement letter as possible. Fellows and residents may feel they are being too demanding and possibly alienating their future bosses by doing this—and they may be correct in some circumstances. But in my opinion, a hiring official unwilling to commit to details in writing is someone who most likely will cause you to regret in fairly short order your decision to accept the position. Contract terms can, of course, allow for flexibility (e.g., "four to six months on ICU service and four to six months on consult service, totaling no more than nine months/academic year"), which every chair/chief and most employees will want to have; flexibility is a practical necessity in running and participating in a large department or division. However, nothing will wreck your first year faster than finding out you are so consumed with direct clinical care and burdensome administrative duties that the possibility of a true academic future is non-existent. On-call frequency, total clinical load, number (and locations) of clinics and outreach assignments, expected volume of clinical work per assignment (e.g., number of patients per clinic), administrative expectations (committees, director roles, etc.), and other duties that will consume your time and energy should be as clearly defined as possible before you walk onto campus as an attending physician. Some inside information: agreement letters, which are non-binding, are not limited in content. Don't accept that "we don't put those types of things in letters" if you believe them to be important. You are entitled to a clear and precise description of the job you are accepting.

Below are some thoughts that you may find helpful as you begin your faculty role.

Concentrate on mastering the basics of daily work as soon as possible. Learn who does what, how to get things done quickly, and who can help with specific types of issues. Find out very specifically what is expected of you in your daily roles: how notes are to be written, any mandatory training, what dashboards are being kept on your performance, how the residency wants their evaluations done, etc. Armed with this information, establish good habits early and stick to them. Ask your medical records department to pull charts needing your signature once weekly and religiously show up to complete them. If you must sign notes or dictations electronically, get in the habit of logging in and completing them regularly, perhaps right before you leave at the end of each day. Write your clinical and procedure notes as soon as you complete the service, when your memory of the care is best and you can complete the note with the least total time and effort. Speak to your billing support person, determine the most reliable, easiest way to get your billings turned in promptly, and make this part of your daily routine. Be sure you clearly understand institutional policies and adhere to them strictly. Learn quickly how to request leave, submit re-imbursable expense reports, and adjust your employee benefits to meet your needs.

The advantages of mastering these early are two-fold. First, you won't have to think about them again unless the requirements change, thereby avoiding the risks of delin-quency, policy violations, lapses in insurance coverage, or lost compensation. Second, however, this is an approach that buys you time in the future: while some of your less dis-ciplined colleagues are racing around trying to sign a hun-dred procedure notes to avoid having their staff privileges suspended, you will be home enjoying a nice dinner with your family or working on a project you choose to do. You will also have more control over your time—a key compo-nent of job satisfaction in any field.

Pass your boards. Many new graduate faculty physicians will be taking one or more board-certifying examinations dur-ing their first year. You do NOT want to have to deal with a re-take the next year and have the pressure associated with boards hanging over you while establishing your practice, getting your research going, or building a new program. The idea that you will have "more time to study" if you defer your exam is a malicious, destructive self-deception: every day further away from training reduces your chance of success on boards. Take them, pass them, and move on.

Demonstrate good citizenship. We can almost always find a reason to miss a faculty, department or division meeting, postpone submitting our schedule requests, or to otherwise not complete the seemingly innumerable mundane require-ments of academic life. There is an old saying that "deci-sions are made by those who show up," and this is especial-ly true of your role as a new faculty member. Initially, at least, make it a high priority to be at regular meetings and fulfill the basic expectations of all faculty physicians at your institution. You will have plenty of time later to do otherwise, should you so choose and for whatever reason.

Initiate contact with key individuals. These will include your mentors (see Chapter 5, *Notes on Finding a Mentor*), the secretarial/administrative support staff members assigned to work with you, perhaps vice chairmen or program directors with whom you will have considerable involvement, and others based on your specific job description and academic plans. The IRB/funded programs coordinator, associate dean for faculty development, chief librarian, statistician, computer support person, practice compliance officer, and others are worth a brief personal visit initiated by you. In addition to gaining very practical information efficiently, you are showing these individuals that you value them—an investment with tremendous potential future returns when you might need their help.

Make a comprehensive schedule of your first-year activities. You should know all your clinical assignments, national meeting dates, even regularly recurring committee and work group meetings, within a week or two of your initial arrival. Compose a schedule to define where you have discretionary time, and plan your time-flexible but essential tasks as soon as possible. Activities with long timelines, such as developing a new clinical program or establishing and building your research activities, need to be started early, assuming (as has been my personal observation) these activities will take at least three times as long to complete as you will conservatively estimate initially.

Establish yourself through character, quality, and work ethic. First impressions are hard to erase. Respect is hard-earned and easily lost. Avoid temptations to gossip, complain, and criticize—even with those participating in these very activities in your presence. Deliver on every single duty and activity to which you agreed—even those that turn out to be more difficult, more demanding, and/or less rewarding than you anticipated. Make it obvious you are there to work and do the job, and that you are committed to the success of the institution and that of your colleagues and other employees. Be accountable and keep your word: there is no substitute for being trustworthy and responsible—EVER.

Learn how to communicate effectively with your superiors. This is a complex, very important but rarely discussed area, so we will spend some additional space here to highlight issues and present possible solutions.

We would all like to think our chiefs and chairmen will advise us toward what is best for our careers. In reality, however, with the changes in health care and academic administration, chiefs, chairs, and even deans are really more "middle managers" at most institutions. They have far less control over the currencies of dollars, space, and personnel than in the past, and these limitations will become more extreme as dollars (above all else) drive daily decisions. They also have far less freedom in designing job descriptions for newly hired faculty physicians, as much of this is now dictated by practice or hospital compensation plans or university requirements. Your superiors must satisfy *their* superiors, prevent mass exodus of faculty, retain "high performers" who fill essential or high-profile roles in the department (even if they are high-maintenance and excessively demanding), balance the books, recruit to fill vacancies, and meet various and sundry other demands. With recent changes directed at empowerment of all employees, they are also subject to evaluations from their staff, their colleagues, and others (the "360 degree evaluation" process). Therefore, even the most well-intentioned superior will not always be looking out for your welfare when he or she has a department of 200 physicians or more to direct. If you expect them to do so, expect also to be disappointed.

We all want to be liked, to be accommodating and perceived as "team players." This is fundamental human nature, and not a bad baseline intent overall; however, the most important word you can learn as a new faculty member is "NO." There are several reasons for this. The first is obvious: if you agree to take on everything asked of you by people who truly don't understand (and sometimes don't really care about) your career needs, you will be consumed by these duties, have neither time nor energy to do the foundation work crucial to your future success, and soon become unfocused and disenchanted with your job. The more accommodating, competent, and personable you are, the more likely different people will try to get you to do things for them—especially things no one else has been willing or able to do. Second, and perhaps more subtly, your superiors and others who "ask" you to do things are people first. People under pressure (whether external or self-imposed) want that pressure relieved with as little effort on their part as possible. Those pressures recur, again and again, in the complex environment of academic health centers and medical schools. If someone figures out that when they need an extra weekend or month on service covered, an extra task done or a person to salvage a failing committee, and asking you first will immediately solve their problem, they have no real motivation to do anything but ask you all the time. They will not realize (largely because it is psychologically inconvenient to do so) that they may be making you feel devalued, abused, and perhaps that you were deceived during your recruitment; when your tolerance of this behavior is exceeded, you may quit and deny the institution the rewards of your future contributions. The business world associates this relationship issue as one requiring you to "manage up": in essence, this means that the subordinate employee, and not the person with authority, may be the one most capable of making the best decisions for the organization in specific circumstances.

Another misconception is that always saying yes will somehow endear you to your superiors, and you will reap some nebulous future benefits. This NEVER happens. The "Yes Sir" individuals may get the occasional bone thrown their way, but for the big rewards they are universally passed over. In fact, I firmly believe that being nothing more than a servant to your superiors, obedient to their every whim, makes them respect you less, and see you more as a tool than a colleague. Nobody disrespects these types of individuals more than their superiors—though no one ever tells you that.

So, how is this apparent dilemma solved? The best approach for you will depend upon your personality, but two basic principles apply to most everyone.

First, understand that the best thing you can do for your institution is to be happy, productive, and successful. Many physicians have been denying their own needs and desires (delayed gratification) for so long they have forgotten to appreciate their real value. You are good. Your superiors know you are good (or they wouldn't have hired you). Your contributions will be maximized when you feel valued; when you are spending your energy on projects and activities you enjoy and feel to be important; when you feel you are being treated fairly and with respect; and when you have hope for even better things in the future. Conversely, your contributions will fall short of their potential when you are angry; feel you have been victimized; become bitter; and see only doom and gloom in the future. Also, should you become totally disenfranchised and quit, replacing you will cost anywhere from four-to-six times the money, time and resources that would have been needed to keep you on staff. Therefore, it is NOT selfish to say "no" at appropriate times, but in fact it is your duty to do so.

Second, seek to be respected FIRST (and liked second if you choose). People like you because you meet needs they have—at some point, failing to meet even one need (which always happens eventually in every relationship) kills that affection (the "What have you done for me lately?" syndrome), and all the time and effort you invested in growing their theoretical good will is lost. (If you doubt this, just watch any President's approval rating, which always dips far below the percentage of the votes they received when elected—usually based upon a single event or issue.) Establishing yourself as someone to be respected is accomplished by taking the moral "high road" all the time, particularly in your discussions with your superiors. No chief or chairman can credibly dispute the principles of fairness, justice, equality, and commitment to the stated (traditional) missions of academic health care institutions: quality care, quality education, quality research and scholarship. Frankly, most could not openly deny your need for career development either (particularly so soon after they promised their support during your contract negotiations!). Therefore, prepare irrefutable reasons to justify why you are saying no. Discuss how the excessive clinical time will cost your research development and reduce the likelihood the institution will recover its investment in your career; how these additional duties will place a disproportionate (i.e., unfair) clinical load on you compared to your colleagues, thereby setting a precedent suggesting unjust treatment of new junior faculty members and hurting future recruitment of internal candidates (the "Eat Their Young" principle); how the additional administrative duties are not consistent with the career path your superior approved and said he or she would support—and upon which you are going to be evaluated, regardless of taking on the unplanned work load.

Sometimes admitting your limitations can be effective. State honestly that you have no interest in a particular activity, no experience or background knowledge in the area, perhaps specifically lack a skill believed to be essential for the role, and do not feel you could provide a credible service in that capacity. (Note: don't be susceptible to feigned praise—which is cheap and spread by the truckload in academic centers—through statements that you are underestimating yourself or are the best person in the department for this job, etc.) Constantly refocus any discussions toward the good of the institution, higher principles, and long-term benefits (and consequences). This also shows a level of vision and maturity uncommon among junior faculty physicians and further supports your position.

Another approach is to negotiate. If you are able to fill an immediate but additional need of your organization, use this opportunity to bring up an additional need you have identified for yourself, such as another meeting you wish to attend, or specific weekends your family obligations would make it difficult to work, or a plum additional appointment you do want. If you get something more for the additional work, it may be worth accepting. In chaos lies opportunity.

The extreme situations should also be mentioned here. If additional assignments are becoming habitual, ask to have a formal meeting with your division director or chairman to re-discuss your career plans and role in the department. It may be that there was honest misunderstanding of your initial agreements, and the sooner these can be clarified the better. Also, this request will suggest (without you stating so directly) that the job is not meeting your expectations and that you may be considering alternative employment opportunities. However, no matter how bad things get, don't threaten to leave UNLESS AND UNTIL you are ready to walk out the door. The first time you make this threat but don't carry through (i.e., don't get what you want but don't resign), you will lose all credibility and no longer have this card to play. Moreover, your only future alternative will be to leave, which may occur at a time when you wish you had other choices. You will be perceived as a complainer, malcontent, problem-child, and in all likelihood seal your (negative) fate at that institution by such feigned threats.

So after all these considerations, when should you decline additional work or assignments? Again, specific circumstances will determine the answer to this question. In general, however, anything that you think might materially derail your first-year goals should be avoided. You, of course, should expect to accommodate your colleagues to a degree, just as you would expect them to do for you (again, fairness). But if you find you are doing 50 percent more call than your older colleagues, that others are refusing additional assignments that you are then expected to accept, or realize the protected time that was contractually guaranteed for your academic development is being treated as "available time" by your superiors, remember that you were not hired to personally fix everyone else's problems: your family life, health, and sanity are as important as anyone's in your division or department. In my opinion, the career needs of junior faculty members *exceed* those of their senior colleagues (you have future and potential, not just some years to pass until retirement).

Beware particularly of major new roles that were not discussed in detail during your contract negotiations. I am amazed at how often a director will say "Dr. X, who is joining us next July, could probably be the director of that program," when clearly this was never discussed with the new physician.

Also watch for requests coming from self-appointed surrogates. If someone tells you that he or she was told by your superior to come to you to get something (new and unexpected) done, immediately contact that superior for clarification and explanation; sometimes, that initial conversation never occurred and the messenger is misrepresenting the situation, while other times the superior may indeed have made the suggestion, but done so without considering the ramifications, and will change his or her mind when confronted with facts (or confronted at all).

There also may be roles and duties to which you agreed initially, but that were misrepresented during initial discussions or about which critical details that vary significantly alter the work load and impact of the duty were omitted. These instances can create an untenable situation that must change if you are to be able to remain on faculty. (As an example, I joined a division of 35 physician members at a large state medical school; as an intensive care cardiologist, my clinical load included six months per year attending on the CCU/inpatient services. I wasn't told that half the CCU attending time included half the night and weekend call for the division, and never imagined that the other 34 cardiologists would only share the remaining six months of call. Needless to say my tenure at that institution was short—and exhausting.)

This is a very complicated situation, requiring more negotiation than the other examples discussed previously. To remedy an extreme miscommunication such as this, you will usually need to formally change roles and basically negotiate a new job description. You will have the best chance if you can present a viable alternative, complete with clear evidence of how you will provide additional benefit to the division or department in your new, more survivable, role. It is also wise to present one or more options for covering the duties you would be giving up with the change, with ample consideration for the good of your co-workers in evidence. You may need to take a salary reduction or give up other benefits (such as protected academic time) upon which you were counting to make this work: remember, once you are there you have expended much of your negotiating capital. You may be surprised at the willingness of your chief or chairman to consider seriously an alternate role for you, particularly if you have performed well up to that point. Unfortunately, an acceptable compromise can sometimes not be reached when the differences in expectations are too extreme, and in this case being honest and conveying that you feel you have no alternative but to look for a position elsewhere is the only viable alternative. If at all possible, try to leave on good terms, give as much notice as you can, and try to never speak negatively of your current superiors when interviewing elsewhere.

————————◆————————

A complete discussion of all potential issues and solutions for new faculty is, of course, far beyond the scope of this chapter. Also, issues will differ when starting a new job after some time on faculty at another institution. Those discussed above are just some that I have experienced, observed, or have had conveyed to me by junior physicians at some time over my career. A few, including communication strategies, were specifically requested by my younger colleagues. I have no doubt you will each find other issues that you will need to address during your first year. When dealing with those issues, keep in mind that there will never be substitutes for having a plan, taking personal responsibility for your career and remaining focused, and acting always with integrity. Your first year is the cornerstone of your professional future—be ready to invest heavily to make it be the year you need it to be.

Chapter 8
Notes on CVs and Documentation
(*Recording and Presenting Your Accomplishments*)

When preparing for promotion, tenure, or applying for jobs, speaking opportunities, elected memberships and a host of other activities, you will need to be able to provide a comprehensive summary of your academic activities and sometimes documentation confirming those activities. An academic curriculum vitae (CV) is a must, but other records are also necessary.

CURRICULUM VITAE

Your CV is a structured listing of accomplishments and achievements related to your career. Its goal is to convey information to the reader. Often, the first information people learn about you, including those whom you have never met or of whom you have never heard, is from your CV. It is in part a documentation tool, part a descriptor of your professional career to date, part an advertisement of the professional you are, and perhaps a suggestion of the one you may become. It is used as an initial screening document for projects and jobs you are seeking; by employers looking to recruit; by your supervisor for evaluations; and by committees who will decide if you get promoted, tenured, elected to a competitive position or society, or be invited as a visiting professor or collaborating investigator. An *effective* CV is one of the most important tools needed by an academic physician. It is well worth the time both to compose initially, and to *maintain and update regularly.*

There are many different formats and content recommendations available, including templates produced by search companies, academic institutions, governments and businesses. Generic examples can be found on the web (use a search engine to locate "Sample Academic CV"). Some medical schools and universities have standardized formats for their faculty, while others use computer-based documentation tools that generate CVs in a pre-specified format. In distinction, specialized bio-sketches are required by some organizations, such as NIH; private sector speakers' bureaus; and funding agencies and organizations: these bio-sketches, unlike CVs, are abbreviated, with content and length limitations specified by the organization.

Although there is no universally-accepted format, effective CVs have certain characteristics in common. These include:

What a CV is NOT. A CV is not a biography of your life, nor an opportunity to pen your own eulogy. You might be very proud of having been grammar school valedictorian or co-captain of your high school dart-throwing team. You may want people to know about your personal life, religious activities, philanthropy, hobbies, and social interests because they are very important to you. You may be a proud parent of many successful offspring, and rightfully so. However, very little of this is appropriate for a CV of an academic physician, and inclusion of such information may be viewed negatively by leaders and others expecting to see a "standardized" document—implying you might not understand what a professional CV should be. Also, CVs now are often posted *in toto* on public access web sites, available to anyone with a browser, including those who might find you an easy target for identity fraud—or worse.

A CV is also not a resume—the type of summary often used in other career lines. Literary descriptions of activities, jobs or positions you have held, or other nonprofessional activities, should be limited in, if not excluded from, an academic CV. Those who read your CV will usually understand the implications of a position or activity from its complete title—and if not, they will ask you if they are sufficiently interested. (It is possible you may apply for jobs outside of health care at some point, and a private sector executive could be considering you for a job; in this case, you may need to prepare a second CV, or a true resume, for this unusual situation.)

Professional Presentation. Human impressions always have significant subjective/emotional components, and you definitely want to support the impression that you are a true professional through your CV. Make your CV polished—well organized, thoroughly proof-read, with consistent entry formatting and devoid of conversational language. Use font modifiers sparingly, and then only in accepted ways (i.e., not to make something look important, but rather easier to find). Look at CVs of established academicians, and take note of the details. It may be a good idea to ask a senior colleague to edit your CV at least once.

Standard Content. There is some information needed by a large proportion of potential readers. Your present position with full and complete professional contact information (including fax number and email address); very basic personal information (year and place of birth, citizenship status, and *perhaps* marital status); a chronologic summary of your formal education (including degrees awarded, dates and degree honors); professional credentials (board certifications, USMLE or ECFMG certification [that is, date you passed the final exam; not the dates and scores you obtained on individual steps], medical licenses and status [active or inactive], and special certifications denoting expertise recognized by an organization or government); hospitals where you *presently* hold staff privileges; regional, national and international professional organizations (including your status as a member, affiliate, fellow, etc.); academic history (faculty appointments and school positions, such as program director, division chief, associate chairman, etc.); publications (Books and Chapters, Peer-reviewed Articles, Published Abstracts, Presented Abstracts, and Other [editorials, symposium pieces, web pages, etc.]); Research Grants and Projects; Invited Lectures (excluding those considered part of your regular job); Other Scholarly Accomplishments; Community Service; and special professional recognitions (awards) are all expected content areas for an academic CV. This list also provides a basic structure (subheadings) for organizing your document.

Limited Personal Information. Home address and phone, social security number, medical license numbers, certificate numbers (such as from ABIM, NBME/USMLE, etc.), cell phone number, and other personally-identifiable information should NOT be on your CV (see above). It may be useful to have a separate document with some of this information, which you can use selectively when needed. Also, meetings you attend, CME credits, and additional courses generally do not belong on a CV, except in rare situations where this information identifies unusual but important credentials (e.g., leadership, business management, and other training be-yond the scope of most academic physicians) or an unusual certification (e.g., Certified Physician Executive, Specialist in Clinical Hypertension). Again, a separate document (such as a spread sheet) can be used to organize these, and thus make them easily available when needed (for recertification, license renewal, etc.).

No Listed References. For reasons cited above, your sup-porters may not appreciate having their contact information all over the web. Keep a separate document of your refer-ences and use it when you have a reason to do so (see be-low).

Readability. Make your CV easy to read, and easy to find specific information when needed. Use a reasonable font (11 or 12 point san serif, such as Arial), appropriate spacing, bullets or numbering where helpful, and categories that are easily understandable. Include page numbers (ideally a footer with your name, auto-update date, and page number), and avoid a lot of font modifiers (such as bold, italics, all caps, etc.)—use these to identify section headings (bold or caps), journal names (italics), and your name (bold) among a list of contributing authors or investigators. Too many font modifiers get lost, making everything in bold look the same—and unintentionally subjugating anything not in bold.

Appropriate Length. Avoid the appearance of trying to make your CV longer than necessary. Common belief is that "bigger is better"—but not when it looks like this is the intent. Depending on its length, a few blank lines are acceptable to allow a specific section (such as Publications or Grants and

Research Activities) to begin on a new page; otherwise, try to have each page appear full, and that the number of pages is justified by content. That also means standard one-inch borders and single spacing within individual entries.

Standard Entry Formatting. Use standard formatting for types of entries where a common standard exists. For example, National Library of Medicine (PubMed) formatting for publications is quite standard:

> Jones AB, Smith DE, Brown GH. How to write a curriculum vitae. *N Engl J Med.* 2009;114(8):43-45.

(Keeping information on your CV in such standard entry format also will allow you to cut-and-paste into other documents when needed—a real time saver for later.)

Dates of Activities. Include applicable dates for most activities. A major red flag is noting, for instance, professional organization affiliations listed as if they are active, when the details of your professional history clearly convey this is not the case; an example is having state medical society memberships listed when you haven't lived in that area for decades. Another reason relates to relative contribution—10 years as an IRB member is clearly a greater contribution to your school than a two-year term.

Precise Entries. Some roles are with your medical school, academic department or division; others may be hospital or practice positions. Some extramural activities are specifically regional, while others are national or international. An industry speakers' bureau role is different than that of an industry consultant, which is different than being an investigator in an industry-sponsored clinical trial. Each has different requirements and implications as to the experience you have obtained and its associated level of accomplishment or recognition. Be sure to include, for example, the name of the sponsoring organization when you list an invited lecture; the funding agency or company that supported your research; accurate names of meetings where you presented; the name of the medical school or hospital you served as associate program director; and the date (or at least year) you performed each role.

Titled by Your Name. It's generally unnecessary to put "CURRICULUM VITAE" on top of your CV—there is little chance it will be interpreted as anything else by anyone you really care about. This may be a small point, but *your name* should be at the top of page 1, the first item on *your CV*.

Organized. You should divide information into sections, and, as your CV grows, subsections. Most people do not have time to read a 50-page CV, or to hunt through every line to find out if you hold an active state medical license, are board-certified, or have successfully competed for research funding. Sections allow readers to find key information quickly and efficiently. Sections best parallel university missions (clinical, research, education, administration) and include standard content areas (see above). As your CV grows, subsections will provide additional structure and readability. For example, separating intramural from extramural (or local from regional from national) educational activities or professional organizations is a common approach. Separating your peer-reviewed manuscript publications into original research, reviews, case studies and reports, published abstracts, presented abstracts, and "other" (to include accomplishments such as sponsored symposia or web pages) is also common when you have a large number of listings. If you have worked at more than one medical school, intramural activities can be separated using the school as a delineator.

Find out early if your school or hospital has a particular CV format, required content, or perhaps a documentation tool that you are expected to use. Once you have an initial draft, ask your director or a senior colleague to edit and critique it for you. Be sure to update it regularly, at least every three months or as soon as you have something to add; you do not want to trust your memory, or a pocket calendar or appointment book, with something this important.

ADDITIONAL DOCUMENTS

Some data not appropriate for your CV are still useful to have recorded and organized in printable documents. These include:

Reference List. Your reference list should have your supporters' full names and titles, and complete professional contact information (including email address)—as listed on their business cards. A short statement about their relationship with you is helpful (e.g., research advisor, residency director, attending physician during clinical rotation), so whoever receives your references will know how to weigh their opinions about particular aspects of your professional achievements. Be sure to have asked each individual in advance if he or she will serve as a reference for you, and exclude personal contact information (such as home or cell phone numbers) unless specifically told you are free to use them by your supporter.

Registration and Credential Numbers. Physicians have what seems to be a continually growing list of identifiers: medical licenses, DEA registration, UPIN or NPI numbers, specialty board certificate numbers, employee numbers, membership numbers for professional organizations, dictation and medical record numbers, user names and passwords—the list can seem endless. Having this together, updated regularly and kept in a *secure* location, can save you time when such information is needed.

Continuing Medical Education Credits. Since state licensing authorities, hospital credentials committees, some third party payers, and perhaps your chairman or director may require or expect you to earn a specific number of CME credits on a regular basis, a running electronic table or spreadsheet is easy to update and, again, can save you time and effort in the long run. Name of course or meeting, location and dates held, sponsoring/CME accrediting organization, and number and category of CME credits earned is sufficient detail. It is a good idea to update this document as soon as you return from an activity or receive the CME certificate. Be sure to also keep the hard copy of the official CME certificate (see below).

Work History. State licensing bureaus, federal health care systems, and most hospitals and HMOs now require a detailed work history, verified from original sources, before granting their credentials. Develop and keep updated a continuous chronology of your work history, starting with medical school. Include contact information for each hospital, employer, training program office, etc. Have an explanation of any breaks in employment of a month or more (such as vacation taken between jobs, medical or maternity leave), and list non-family members who can confirm your activities during such times.

Portfolio. Many of your accomplishments do not belong in a CV, though they clearly deserve credit when being considered for academic promotion, or assessing experience or expertise in a given field. Portfolios are detailed, organized records of your activities within a given "mission," such as education or administration. They include more specifics than is appropriate for a CV—for example, an educator portfolio might include individual intramural lectures or workshops, details as to audience composition, number of attendees, course evaluations, etc. Similarly, an administrator portfolio might include descriptions of responsibilities, activities, and achievements associated with individual work groups, directorships, committee chairmanships, etc.—much like a resume used in the business world. If your goals include high-level positions in educational or hospital/clinical administration, a portfolio is a must for career advancement.

OTHER DOCUMENTATION

From as early in your career as possible, you should create and maintain files of materials that document your achievements and contributions. Promotion committees, your department and school, future employers, hospital credentialing offices, and even state licensing agencies may require documentation of one or more aspects of your professional accomplishments.

Keep a copy of each annual faculty evaluation you receive, and the faculty activity summary you submit for these evaluations. If you present an abstract, keep a copy AND the program for the meeting where you presented. Ask for a thank-you letter or email if you give lectures for another department or school, or serve as a preceptor for a student in a health-related field. Copies of hand-outs and printed slides, rotation outlines, hospital policies, or other works you write should be kept in your files. Keep letters from professional societies appointing you to leadership positions or committees, as well as the thank-you letters you receive when your terms are completed. Keep letters appointing you to hospital committees, work groups, task forces, and other official intramural roles. If you receive an annual summary of fellow, resident or student evaluations of your teaching, hold on to these too. Copies of your publications, web pages, editorial board listings, and even newspaper announcements all provide helpful documentation. Ask the journals for which you review for a letter confirming the number of manuscripts you reviewed for the year (some with more sophisticated electronic submission systems can print out a confirmation upon request), and if you receive a thank-you email for a review, print and file it. Keep your CME certificates, and if possible a copy of the sessions you attended or content of the course—some certifications require a requisite number of CME credits in a topic area for eligibility. Keep records from previous jobs in all these categories also, as these may be needed for academic promotion at your present school.

Of course, you should maintain easy access to all your official documents. Your medical school diploma, training certificates, board certifications, professional college fellowships (e.g., F.A.C.P.), active medical license and DEA certificate are frequently needed for various purposes. If you choose to mount the originals for display, make a master copy first (and perhaps even have it notarized) that you can then photocopy for additional copies at any time.

———————◆———————

We live in a world that believes that "if it isn't in writing, it didn't happen," Documentation is necessary for YOUR career, and is your responsibility—for only you will suffer from its absence or insufficiency. An academic physician's documentation starts with an updated, professionally formatted CV, but includes other documents and materials that verify your accomplishments. You work hard and contribute much—be sure you are credited for all that you do.

Chapter 9
Notes on Time Management

You have likely already concluded that your most precious resource during your academic career will be neither money nor knowledge, but time (with which you can obtain money, knowledge, and most other things). Most of us chose to pretend that the conclusion of our training programs would end the continuous time pressure we had experienced since starting medical school many years ago; within the first few days of our first job, however, we quickly realize time pressures become even greater at the staff physician level. As faculty members, we now have responsibilities for effectively supervising our trainees and students, additional requirements for billing and clinical/regulatory documentation, and a perceived greater need for certainty in our clinical work—as we no longer have the safety net of a supervising attending following behind us. Moreover, the diverse demands on our time can only be expected to grow as financial, regulatory, quality of care, and other needs expand in directions requiring more production from, and less support for, each of us.

At most institutions, however, there are a few people who seem consistently more productive than most: they appear to be immune to the time pressures other faculty members are experiencing, always managing to broaden their scope of influence, writing and performing research, growing their extramural reputations, and otherwise producing valuable academic products with remarkable regularity. Generally we attribute their success to innate ability, genetically-determined ambivalence to biological needs such as sleep, and/or a psychopathological commitment to their careers that ultimately compromise their families, social skills, sanity and perhaps coronary circulation. Having been identified as one of these individuals, and having known several others over the past 30 years, I can assure you that effective time management is a skill that can be learned. Just as you learned efficiency in much of your clinical work, so too can these skills be applied successfully to academic pursuits and scholarly activities.

Here are some ideas that you can apply to improve your time management skills and boost your academic productivity (without compromising your health and family life in the process). You are probably familiar with some of them:

Try to "touch paper" only once. We all have stacks of paper—articles, hand-outs, references, advertisements, memos—piled up somewhere in our homes or offices that we thought we would "get to" at some point. Electronic communications, mostly emails, have joined company with these other stacks, and often become yet another pile of items "to be addressed." Most of the materials we have saved for review at a later time are never seen again. Deadlines pass, opportunities are lost, and often we are paying late fees, receiving delinquency notices from our chairmen or hospital administrators, or finding we have insulted a colleague by not addressing their communications in a timely fashion. The majority of routine communications can be addressed definitively in a matter of seconds to minutes; a small number will take a bit of time to complete, and a few represent large time commitments. Try to deal with each communication as soon as it is received, make the necessary decision, and THEN file or discard the paperwork as appropriate. Certainly you will receive some number of items requiring more time—and for this, create a task list that you habitually complete on a regular basis (e.g., Friday afternoons before leaving for the weekend, or your regular Tuesday afternoon non-clinical time).

Never leave your mail unopened. Any un-reviewed communication has the potential of a limited time window during which it can be easily addressed, and every one that requires a response or action on your part most certainly has a finite period for resolution. People use email boxes differently, but keep your in-box clear of unopened messages. The longer they sit there, the easier it is to procrastinate when other demands on your time seem more urgent—and soon you will have dozens (and sometimes hundreds) of individual communications to review, make decisions upon, and sometimes have your email accounts inactivated due to excessive volume!

Set early personal deadlines and stick to them. One of the few things we can all be sure about is that there is little if anything about which we can be sure. The potential to have our best-planned schedules set awry by external influences beyond our control has become standard operating procedure. Yet, try as we might, anything from a flat tire to a surprise Joint Commission survey, from an unexpectedly acutely ill patient to a resident who takes emergency leave can derail our best-laid plans. Your defense here is to set deadlines for completing necessary tasks in advance of the actual "drop-dead" due date. Lead time should vary with activity, with small projects such as mandatory review of a 30-minute continuing education module earning a few days of lead time, while a grant application (with a four- to six-month schedule for completion) needing a personal lead-time deadline of a few weeks to a month in advance. The key for success in this approach is sticking to the deadlines you set for yourself, just as if they were the externally-determined deadlines. It takes some discipline initially, but the benefits in productivity (and stress reduction in never missing a true deadline) quickly add value to your life and existence. I have known no "high performers" who do not employ this technique regularly.

Use technology—don't let it use you. I have lived long enough to see technological advancements, from the automatic answering machine and radio pagers to cell phones, internet-capable personal computers and PDAs, enter our lives, all with the promise of saving us time and effort and improving our lives. They never have. Constant availability via electronics has reduced the threshold for others to seek contact with us, and has expanded expectations for immediate responses, disseminated responsibility, and added demands for service well beyond the ability of most humans to meet. Our defense often becomes nonspecific, answering no emails, turning off cell phones, blocking text messaging, etc.—so we might actually secure uninterrupted time to accomplish those tasks we hold important—such as speaking with a patient about a dismal prognosis, writing an abstract, or dining with our families on a day off. I readily admit this phenomenon has generational considerations, and younger physicians who grew up with more advanced technology may find the negative impact of 24/7/365 availability to anyone who can find our email addresses or smart phone numbers less intrusive, but such effort does not change the fact that we all have duties that require our uninterrupted attention to complete successfully.

Know your personal performance psychology and biorhythms. Some of us are night people, while some are morning people. Some are sprinters, while others perform best at a regular consistent pace. Some need totally undisturbed time, devoid of distractions, to complete certain tasks, while others can seemingly multi-task with no compromise of performance. Some work best under pressure (or feel they do), while others find looming deadlines so distracting they abandon activities to avoid these feelings. As discussed in Chapter 2, *Notes on Career Planning*, a thorough understanding of yourself may be the most important knowledge you can acquire to assure a successful academic career, and in this area of work performance that knowledge is particularly valuable. As best you can, try to schedule your work to fit optimally with your personal performance characteristics. This is a somewhat complex concept with which you are probably familiar; raising this familiarity to deliberate planning can be very effective in enhancing your productivity.

Look for "multiple-credit" projects and activities. (See Chapter 6, *Notes on Choosing Projects.*) This is more of a strategic than tactical principle, but still worth mentioning. The more birds you can kill with fewer stones, the more time you will have to do things other than throwing stones at birds. Choosing projects and activities that fulfill multiple needs in your career development can improve your efficiency by requiring you to complete fewer total projects overall. Faculty members with the thickest CVs learned this early—so should you!

Find ways to use down time. No matter how busy we think we are, we all have small bits of down time—waiting for a meeting to start (or maybe sitting in a meeting), awaiting lab results or an x-ray to be completed, sitting in the dentist's waiting room or an automobile service center, enduring flight delays, sitting in traffic in a taxi or in the stands at a little league game when your child isn't playing. If you are ever able to track this time, you will be amazed at how many hours per week pass without useful content—not by your choice, but by circumstances beyond your control. You can usually identify these times by your frustration level—when high, time is being wasted. We have a number of portable projects—articles to read, lectures to outline, schedules to construct, ideas to organize. Start to make it a habit to always have something with you that you could work on—for five to ten minutes, or for an hour or more. This approach will not only increase your effective work time, but could do wonders at controlling your blood pressure.

Maximize your use of standardized (reusable) forms and templates. You learned as an intern how to become efficient at similar, repeated tasks—organizing your histories and physicals, getting your lab results, and presenting cases. These same organizational skills can be applied to academic activities. For example, systematic review articles use a standard format—easily saved on a word processor for the next review, and the next. If you submit manuscripts to one or two journals frequently, each will have standard requirements for content and formatting of title pages, cover letters, conflict of interest disclosures, etc. Make a template that you can reuse and complete in a fraction of the time needed to compose an original from scratch. A PowerPoint template that is simple, adaptable, and organized can reduce the time needed to create a traditional lecture by half. These are just a few examples.

Always remember: "Perfect" is the mortal enemy of "Good Enough." We all like to do our best. At times, we really need to. But striving for perfection when perfection is not valued beyond good can be a tremendous waste of time and effort. There isn't a grant proposal, manuscript, lecture, or administrative document that you couldn't make better with more time and effort. But why? The goal of a grant proposal is to obtain funding—so it needs to be only "good enough" to compete successfully. A lecture is intended to convey certain information to a target audience; if that can be done with simple slides, what benefit is there to cines, flying text, and dozens of additional references? If a policy paper spells out the necessary information in an organized and clearly understandable form, do hours of literary polishing add anything to the outcome? This is a key concept mastered by those high producers. Identify the need, then meet it. Done. Next case.

Plan strategically: Employ advance preparation whenever possible. Military people know the importance of advance preparation, anticipation, and planning better than most others. They train, foresee contingencies, look at probabilities, and prepare alternatives for every imaginable battle scenario. Academic physicians can do the same—and often do so without realizing it. For example, if you regularly attend on an inpatient hospital service supervising and teaching residents and fellows, you have a pretty good idea of key topics you will want them to learn during the month— perhaps based on deficits elsewhere in their training, or driven by your particular patient population. Yet it can be difficult (and sometimes impossible) to do all the personal teaching to cover these topics comprehensibly each month. Efficient teachers will have prepared, in advance, variations of talks on their favorite topics: a two- to five-minute version (very basics needed for safe patient care); a 10- to 15-minute version (adding depth but not a comprehensive review); and a longer, perhaps 50-minute version for the classroom. If you supervise a telescoped team (with members ranging from third-year medical students through third-year fellows), you likely need different versions appropriate to the different learner levels. Having full lectures (slide sets) or review articles saved on your PDA can also be useful, allowing you to spend less time speaking but assuring your trainees have the detailed information they will need.

Another aspect of advanced planning is use of a comprehensive (probably electronic) calendar. Since your time is used for all types of activities, it is best to use a calendar that allows you to put in all the things that consume your time—and to use it that way. Some activities recur regularly (monthly division meetings, grand rounds, quarterly committee meetings), and others can be entered months or even years in advance (national professional meetings, lectures you will be giving, etc.). Reminders can be set minutes, hours, or days/weeks in advance. Knowledge truly is power here. The more comprehensive your calendar, the more control you will have over your time. You can group elective meetings, combine tasks, use geography to your advantage (multiple tasks at a single site or building over a short time period), and reduce down time with thoughtful scheduling using a comprehensive calendar.

Avoid both unrealistic expectations and falsely low estimates of what you can do with your available time. *(*See Chapter 2, *Notes on Career Planning*.) Your academic career is a triathlon, not a hundred-meter dash. If you continually find yourself working at (or beyond) your perceived limits, you will exhaust yourself and lose the race. Conversely, if you avoid running, cycling, and swimming whenever possible, you cannot win. As early as practical, start to formulate a strategy consistent with your abilities and goals. Thoughtfully review this strategy periodically and adjust the parts that aren't working the way you want them to work for you. For example, if you want to develop your career as a clinician, educator, and writer, proportion your time and effort to keep a balance of scholastic activities in these areas. Don't commit to three large education projects at the same time, then try to squeeze in some writing and clinical skill development in addition—you will be bleeding your personal time with the expected detriment and potential burn out. Although you want to seize good opportunities when they arise, you also want to be alive to see them to completion—hopefully with your health and personal life intact.

Develop other effective time management habits. The tactics described above are only a few examples of ways you can improve your academic efficiency and produce more for less. You will identify more time management habits, particularly applicable to your needs and abilities, as you begin to apply the concept of *"continuous efficiency improvement"* to your academic activities—the way you have to other aspects of your life. Look for opportunities to spend two minutes each day clearing a recurring responsibility from your desk. Signing medical records is a good example: rather than letting them pile up and having to urgently spend hours some evening signing a hundred charts to avoid negative consequences (such as having your hospital privileges suspended), devoting a very small amount of time each day to reviewing your charts makes the task less formidable (and keeps your administrators happy). Try to review your calendar and schedules with some regularity— you may be able to adjust a few flexible activities and "create" blocks of time you can use for more complex tasks and projects. Learn not to say "yes" every time you are asked to do something; a polite "let me think about that and get back to you" may save huge amounts of time otherwise lost to unnecessary activities. Actively seek to identify more opportunities. Try to get more efficient every day.

———————◆———————

Time is the only truly limited quantity in our academic lives. The more wisely you spend it, the more you will obtain from it.

Chapter 10
Notes on Part-Time Faculty Positions

At some point, you will accept the reality of a 24-hour day, and seek to accomplish all you can in the time available. While organization and wise choices can help you make the most of those hours, there is no way to create more time—so choices on how those precious hours are allocated between work and the other things that fill your life will need to be made. Some academic physicians decide the hours spent elsewhere are more precious to them than the hours spent (and dollars earned) at work, and will explore the option of part-time employment.

As with all important issues, this should be an informed, thoughtful decision. The goal of this chapter is to provide a logical process for considering part-time employment, and suggest ideas for negotiating the specifics with your intended employer. While practical issues are discussed, the benefits of a reduced work week are often intangible. Regardless of the financial and professional sacrifices involved, many academic physicians find that part-time employment provides the best of both worlds—allowing for a fulfilling career along with a meaningful life outside of work. Following are questions/issues you should address.

What is motivating your desire for reduced work hours?
The desire for balance between personal and professional life is increasingly felt by younger physicians, particularly those who are the primary caregiver to children or aging parents. The key questions to ask are what you actually need to achieve balance, and then whether part-time employment offers the best way to satisfy your needs. A sudden life change, such as the birth of a child, personal or family illness, or divorce often precipitates a desire for more time outside work. While it is normal for these events to realign your values, make sure your decision is well-contemplated and not reactionary. Moving to part-time employment should be complementary to your life plan, not a change you feel forced to make.

If your only reason for considering part-time employment is to reduce stress caused by heavy, broad responsibilities, have you considered alternative solutions? Do you have inadequate child care, elder care or home help, so that hiring a maid, sitter, home organizer or office assistant would let you function more efficiently in your many roles? Do you have medical or personal leave that would allow you to spend more time at home or with loved ones? Could you alter your work hours to better accommodate the diverse demands of your life, and perhaps do some of your work from home using computer/web communications? Are modifiable work-related factors, such as inadequate nursing or clerical support, influencing your decision? Is it possible that guilt and/or untreated depression are contributing factors? Alternative solutions could prove superior to conversion to part-time employment in these and some other circumstances.

Are you dissatisfied with your career path? Working less will not change your being dissatisfied, but part-time employment may provide a mechanism to achieve the different outcome of redirecting your professional life. This change may provide an opportunity to pursue additional education or training, apply for another type of position, or work in a different setting or facility. You should consider the reasons for your dissatisfaction, and perhaps explore alternatives, before deciding to go part-time.

If after examining these questions you conclude you are satisfied with your career but need to gain personal time, then reducing your professional workload may be a logical choice. Additional issues you should first address include economic and professional considerations.

Economic Considerations. Before approaching your employer, do your homework. Have a good idea of how to structure your proposed new position, and how this position should be compensated. The reduction in gross income is obvious, but part-time employment may also alter your eligibility for benefits, incentive pay, and retirement fund contributions. Some institutions only provide benefits to people who work a minimum of half-time, while some others have complex rules that you will need to read to believe. You should ensure that you have plans for health, life, and malpractice insurance, as well as a financial plan for retirement (pension or personal contributions), and a clear understanding of what extra costs you may incur as a result of your new, less-than-full-time status.

Many work-related expenses remain constant whether you are employed full-time or part-time. A monthly parking fee will not be adjusted to fit your less frequent visits to the hospital or medical school. Many daycare centers also charge a set fee regardless of how many hours your children are actually there. If your new schedule will have you working fewer hours per day but the same number of days each week, your costs for commuting and business clothing will not fall.

Professional Considerations. Part-time faculty will likely spend more years at junior ranks, since it typically takes longer to reach the milestones necessary for academic promotion. Your institution may have a set time period for promotional review regardless of your work hours, particularly if you remain in a tenure track—which can limit your chances of staying at that institution indefinitely (the "up or out" principle)—while others may allow a hiatus ("stopping the clock") for a finite period of time for special circumstances such as child or elder care. Research funding opportunities (both intramural and extramural) are often restricted to full-time academic physicians, or to those with a minimum ongoing percent employment; because more types of grants are available to junior faculty, part-time employment early in your career could have more substantial repercussions for clinician investigators and physician scientists than for clinicians and clinician educators. Professional "burn-out" appears to be less of a threat to part-time academic physicians, and many continue to publish and produce scholarly output while working part-time. Because an academic career can last decades, people who choose part-time employment for a temporary period of time may "catch up" in terms of productivity in later years—though not doing so is a very real risk, and is in fact the rule rather than the exception.

With this knowledge in hand, you can then pursue part-time employment options. These are questions to consider:

- **Do you desire a temporary or long-term change in employment status?** A natural end point for part-time work may exist, particularly when caring for a young child or family member, or when recovering from a personal illness. If you are seeking a different lifestyle, however, a more permanent restructuring of your career will be needed. Some institutions that do not normally have part-time physician employees may consider a special request for a limited period, particularly if you have worked there for some time and performed well; some may not, while others may have one or more of the options below available.

- **What options does your institution have for part-time employment?** Part-time employment is anything less than full time, and descriptions vary across institutions and medical specialties. Some organizations and practices may have defined an FTE (full-time equivalent) based on a model different than the 40-hour work week, perhaps resulting from the advice of a practice consultant, or regulations and requirements of your employer's parent organization. Other institutions may not have even contemplated, much less committed to, a formal definition of an FTE. Given that most physicians work more than 40 hours per week, even individual physicians' definitions will vary. It is within this setting you will need to identify (or propose) a part-time employment model, which can get very complicated. Institutions that employ a production-based compensation model may be more amenable to defining a part-time schedule, though this is not always true. Logic seems to dictate that a 0.75 FTE position, for example, would require 25% less work, including on-call, inpatient service, outpatient clinics, and educational contributions. However, this cannot be assumed (the 25% time you give up may include all of your previous nonclinical time). As you gather information, ask very specific questions about these critical components of your work expectations.

Another possible option is "job-sharing," which typically involves two or more employees sharing the work load (and salary) of a single full-time faculty physician; though most often these are evenly split positions, other options (75%/25%) may also be possible. Job-sharers may, for example, each care for half of a full panel of clinic patients, divide inpatient rotations, and split call. Such a distribution of duties requires careful negotiation, clear documentation, and flexibility. You will need to be able to trust and work cooperatively with your job partner(s) to make this model work. Realistically, you should expect to be contacted during your off-duty time with patient issues that require your immediate attention when engaged in a job-share arrangement. Also remember that the others "sharing" this job likely have their own special needs and expectations (which is why they too are taking this path) that you will need to accommodate with the same flexibility and consideration you desire for yourself.

Another model is "per diem," work "by the day" or "as needed." This option allows considerable flexibility, but usually provides minimal non-salary benefits, often results in unpredictable schedules (and total compensation, based on rate and work availability), and usually has an employment duration limited by contract. Academic health centers rarely use this structure beyond filling short-term, unexpected staffing needs, and when used, they virtually never include paid protected time for academic pursuits. Per diem work should best be viewed as a temporary way to secure some income, but is not a final career path for most academicians.

- **Which negotiation issues may be helpful?** When you are asking for something, you need to offer something in return. Although a few organizations, such as government medical centers, may afford you the "right" to reduce your work time, they are the exception to the rule. Part-time faculty physician jobs can create myriad problems for your institution: they may affect their fiscal reports and accreditation status for training programs; require a considerable amount of administrator time for documentation, contract approvals, human resources processing, etc.; and may offer little perceived benefit to a well-staffed academic health center. Therefore, you should be prepared to offer some specific services your employer will find of value to motivate them to look favorably on your request. Such offerings are as varied as the institutions and physicians involved, but usually with a little investigation (or perhaps a minute of reflection) you can identify one or more acute or chronic needs that you may be able to satisfy in a part-time role. A few examples include a specialized but low-volume clinic/office service; guaranteed days performing specific needed operations or procedures; working on a traditionally less desirable inpatient unit; or accepting an administrative role to build a needed program, resolve a long-standing deficiency, or run an unpopular but needed committee. Anything you are prepared to offer increases your chances of getting the part-time job you seek, and every agreement is in fact a negotiation.

- **What other options might you consider?** If your need for part-time employment is predictably limited, you may also consider working for another employer (perhaps a corporation or government institution) and ask to keep your academic appointment (without compensation) at your medical school or academic health center. Not every institution will offer such an arrangement, but with the ongoing need for part-time (volunteer) faculty to meet the teaching needs of growing medical school classes and GME training programs, this can often be a viable option. This approach will only be available to non-tenure track faculty members, and the contribution of these years to "time at rank" for later promotion may be unpredictable. However, it could offer opportunities for you to continue to build your CV/portfolio and maintain options for ongoing academic pursuits such as clinical trials, teaching, educational administration, and other collaborations.

————————◆————————

No matter the financial or professional cost, part-time employment will definitely offer more of the most precious commodity of all: time. Part-time employment can provide a rewarding experience both personally and professionally, but you need to understand all the relevant issues to make a well-informed decision about this career option.

Chapter 11
Notes on Pregnancy and Early Child Care
(*for the Female Physician*)

Choosing to Have a Family

The age at which most young academic physicians embark on their career parallels the time when one may decide to begin a family. For the female physician who thinks she may want to become pregnant, the perfect time to become a mother simply does not exist. At an earlier career stage, you have less control over your schedule and less income. At a later career stage you may have more financial security and job flexibility but your body may be less amenable to pregnancy. Alternatively, it may be easier to schedule maternity/paternity leave from a training program than a private practice group. In some instances, nature does not give you the option of letting you make your own decision, but makes it for you. There is no surprise quite like finding out you or your significant other is pregnant!

On a more practical side, it is very important to revisit the maternity leave policy of your employer when considering pregnancy. Notice the word "revisit": this policy should be closely examined before signing a contract by anyone who has the potential to become pregnant. You should also review your health insurance policy regarding pregnancy and dependent coverage. Some insurance policies require pre-authorization before delivery of the infant to cover the mother's hospital stay. Others will only allow the addition of the infant to this policy if notified within 30 days of delivery. You do not want to discover these things outside the notification time window.

Managing the Pregnancy

Pregnancy is not a benign condition. Prenatal care was not invented to give obstetricians or family practitioners something to do. Despite your busy schedule, you will need to make time for rest, proper nutrition, and doctor's visits. When choosing your obstetrician, it may serve you well to consider the ease with which you can make your follow-up appointments—or an emergent one. Many pregnant physicians are uneasy about utilizing prenatal care affiliated with their own practice or institution; however, this is likely a very convenient option. Remember the people who work with you are professionals and will give you the same respect you would give them. Not only will getting to appointments at your own institution be easier, employees often receive discounts which, when added to insurance coverage, can substantially reduce your out-of-pocket expenses for the pregnancy. If you are at an academic institution, these doctors manage the most complicated pregnancies—so if you do experience a problem, you are already in the right place.

And if you haven't given up impractical shoes, now is the time. Your feet require more support during pregnancy. Do yourself a favor and invest in a pair that allows room for third trimester swelling.

When to Share your Good News
Traditionally, expectant parents wait until the second trimester to announce the pregnancy. The rationale for this delay is that most miscarriages occur in the first trimester, so waiting avoids having to discuss a miscarriage with others. Given that you work with other health care professionals, they will probably know you are pregnant before you tell them. The change in diet, the fatigue, and the frequent trips to the restroom are dead giveaways!

When to share your good news is certainly a matter of personal preference, but an early official notification will make it easier on the people with whom you work. Patient care and teaching responsibilities will have to go on without you, and planning for a prolonged absence can be difficult for those who manage such details. If you are a resident or fellow, your program director will thank you for providing early notice, and he or she should follow your lead on telling others.

Planning for the Baby
Finding appropriate childcare for your infant is essential not only to allow you to work, but also to accommodate your best on-the-job performance. Nothing is more distracting

than worrying about the safety and well-being of your child when working. Because of this, many hospitals and academic centers have their own on-site childcare centers which can be convenient and nurturing options for employees. If you do not have this option, the search for childcare cannot be done too early. Infant rooms have long waiting lists, and finding in-home care can be challenging. Even if you are fortunate to have a relative who can provide care, illness and infirmity can strike without warning. You should locate several potential options to ensure you will have care in place once the baby arrives.

Co-workers are often very helpful in supplying referrals to day care centers, but you will also want to conduct your own research. If possible, visit the centers on at least two occasions, at different times of the day. This will not only allow you to meet multiple caregivers, but also evaluate traffic conditions. Certainly the safety and well-being of your child is your top priority, but the impact of your drive for drop-off and pick-up could affect your working hours. For that reason, you should also consider the day care center's hours of operation and days of closure. Centers also vary on the age at which they will accept infants. While most centers will accept infants after they have received their first series of immunizations, some do not take infants younger than three months old.

Despite your accomplishments at this point in your life, you most likely do not have the experience or skill set to choose child care on your own. Having a knowledgeable person visit the center and/or interview the potential caregiver either with you or separately can provide invaluable insight. In general, you want to find gentle caregivers and an organized center director. You should sit down with the center director and feel comfortable asking candid questions. Be sure to inquire about the infant room schedule, teacher-to-infant ratio, and how children are transitioned into new rooms. Some centers require infants to be transitioned from part-time into full-time care, which translates into you not being able to work a full-time schedule initially.

Financial Issues

Neither children nor money grow on trees. The tax break you receive for having a child does not nearly cover their expenses. As you evaluate your monthly budget, you should anticipate increased expenditures for medical bills, childcare, and diapers (don't under-estimate this last expense!). The medical bills do not end with prenatal care and delivery. Your infant will have a series of check-ups and immunizations. (If immunizations are not covered by your insurance plan, you should plan on getting them at your local health department.) Check to see if your, or your spouse's, employer has flexible medical and/or dependent care reimbursement accounts. Do not assume you are not eligible if you are a resident or fellow at the time of your child's birth. If you are an employee of a hospital or university, you are very likely entitled to the benefits of other employees.

Remember to budget for your child's education. The sooner you start saving, the better. Physicians early in their careers often delay saving for their children's college. Every year your child gets older is one less year you have to save for college. Meet with your banker or financial advisor and ask about college saving plans. You would be surprised how much a little investment now can grow in 18 years.

Returning to Work

Returning to work after having a baby is difficult on many levels. Your clothes do not fit, you haven't slept properly in weeks, and your hormones have not settled into a predictable pattern. You may not have given much thought to your professional life since you went into labor. Also, the emotional toll of leaving an infant in day care for the first time can be more difficult than anticipated. However, there are things you can do before your first day back on the job to make going back to work less of a shock to your system.

If you are using a day care center, plan to visit the center with your infant several days before you actually return to work. Bring all of the supplies that you are required to bring (usually a long list and a full trunk-load) before your first official day. Spend some time with your baby's caregivers to increase your comfort level before leaving them with your precious bundle of joy. There is nothing wrong with having a family and a fulfilling career, so allow yourself to enjoy both without guilt.

Pull out your work clothes and see what fits: have a week's worth of professional attire ready before returning to work. Shopping for clothes will only be more difficult after you return to work, so plan ahead on this one. If you are nursing your baby and plan to use a breast pump, you want to make sure you have clothes that are amenable to this. The dress that zips up in the back may not be ideal.

If you have an office, go there before you start back and stock up on supplies. The less you have to carry in every day, the easier it will be for you. You may find it easier to eat breakfast at work than at home. If you have access to a freezer, consider storing several frozen dinners for quick lunches. Nursing mothers need to have an extra shirt, laboratory coat, breast pads, and milk storage bottles. If you are nursing, make sure you have access to snacks and plenty of water.

Take a minute to remind yourself why you embarked on a career in medicine in the first place. Reaffirming that your job is an important part of your life will help you get through this difficult transition. Your job is an investment in you and in your child's future. A female physician will always be able to provide adequately for her family—there is no reason for guilt. Embrace your work as much as you hug your baby. They are both important to you.

Notes on Nursing
Nursing a baby is truly the one thing you can give your child that no one else can. No one can deny the health benefits or cost-effectiveness of breast milk. But it is not a cake walk. Being the only source of food for a baby is a huge job and requires your commitment to getting proper rest, hydration, and nutrition. Once you return to work, toting an electric breast pump can lead to shoulder and back pain. Finding time to pump can be difficult, particularly if you perform long procedures, work with critically ill patients, or do shift work. However, nursing is a wonderful gift to your child and if you truly want to do it, you should. If you have decided that you

are completely committed to breastfeeding your baby, then you should communicate this decision to your co-workers. Your supervisors must support you and your staff and colleagues should be willing to incur minor inconveniences themselves, if necessary, to allow you to do this. If you have a flexible schedule, many daycare centers allow and encourage you to visit during the day to nurse your baby.

If you notice that your milk supply is diminishing, you will need to increase your fluid intake. If you can spend one day a week allowing your baby to nurse on demand, you should maintain a good supply, though your schedule may not allow this. Many physician mothers find that despite their best intentions, they are unable to pump milk frequently enough to completely meet their infants' needs. Do the best you can. While breast milk is superior to formula, formula is a completely appropriate means of nourishing an infant. Many women provide as much milk as they can but supplement with formula. If you have a predictable schedule, you can nurse while with your infant, leave formula with your caregivers, and ditch the breast pump.

If you find the work of breastfeeding is more than you can handle, don't feel guilty. Starving your infant is a bad decision; giving them formula is not. You have to take care of yourself in order to take care of your baby and your patients. Being a physician and a parent involves a lot of compromise—this will be the first of many. You can be good at both, but probably not perfect at either. Find your comfort zone and allow yourself to enjoy both of these important and fulfilling aspects of your life.

————————◆————————

Pregnancy and early child rearing is a major life-changing experience, accompanied by significant costs but also great joys. Like most important things in life, forethought and advance planning, accompanied by careful decision-making, can help smooth the integration of your roles as a physician and a mother.

Chapter 12
Notes on Attending
Your First Professional Meeting

Academic physicians attend meetings of professional organizations with variable frequency, but everyone has a "first time," and a little planning can help optimize the experience.

Meetings are different than courses, where attendees are there to learn in a classroom or workshop setting. Meetings vary in size and venue—from regional meetings and smaller national organizations generally having a few hundred attendees and held at a hotel or resort, to international symposia with upwards of 40,000 attendees and held at large convention centers. They will typically have different types of sessions—reviews, debates, original research (platforms and posters), state-of-the-art and named lectures, hands-on workshops, point-counterpoint presentations, case-based discussions, and others.

Large national/international meetings can be overwhelming at first—some may have 30 or more simultaneous sessions scattered throughout an enormous building. They generally have a broad group of attendees, with multiple simultaneous presentations and many choices of sessions to attend.

Your first meeting may also involve your delivery of a presentation—a poster, plenary, platform, or case presentation. The following points offer some practical advice that can make your first meeting go more smoothly and maximize your experience. These comments will focus on large meetings and include considerations if you are giving a presentation.

Packing and Advance Preparation

Pack appropriate attire. The typical dress code for most scientific meetings is "business casual." Individual meeting rooms can be cool even in the warmest climates, or uncomfortably warm even in the dead of winter. Flexibility in dress and comfort are important, while assuring to maintain a professional appearance. Some convention centers are so large as to require a twenty-minute brisk walk between sessions, so comfortable shoes are also a necessity. Be sure to bring enough outfits with you for the entire length of the meeting.

Useful items. A shoulder bag may be provided with your registration materials, but it never hurts to bring one with you. You may have abstract books, large printed programs, and educational/informational materials you will obtain at the meeting and exhibits, as well as a note pad and pen. You may also choose to carry some personal items with you, particularly if your hotel is a bus ride from the convention center: medications, travel umbrella, business cards, tissues, snacks or a drink. Some meetings have sessions starting as early as 5:30 am and others ending as late as at 9:00 pm, so these days can be long and busy; running back to your hotel room to get an aspirin could cost you hours and force you to miss some of the most valuable sessions. Carrying change and small bills for vending machines, tips, taxis, etc. is a good idea. Don't forget any essentials, such as your cell phone/PDA charger, medications, a sweater or jacket, pen and pad, and business cards.

Plan your itinerary. With so many choices, planning the itinerary of sessions you wish to attend can be challenging. Many organizations provide a web-based filtering tool— entering some personal interest data that prunes down the recommended sessions for you to consider. Others will group sessions by topic (e.g., heart failure), discipline (e.g., clinical cardiology) or format (e.g., original research). Increasingly, meeting planners are providing PDA-downloadable agendas, and most provide a pocket-sized, abbreviated program in hard copy. Regardless, it is always wise to plan ahead, prioritize your sessions, and generally have a back-up choice for any given time slot (some are presented in small rooms with limited seating). Also, look at the map of the convention center—this is typically available on web sites or in the main program book—so you can estimate the time required to walk from one session to the next, which may be considerable. Be aware that some sessions may be held at remote sites, such as other hotels in the area, rather than at the main convention center. If you will be traveling from hotel to convention center by shuttle bus, get your route number and location for pick-up and drop-off in advance from the program.

Also, if you are planning to meet up with old acquaintances, pick a location that is easy to find, specific, and unique (such as the meeting registration desk, or convention center stop for Shuttle Bus #1)—and exchange cell phone numbers in advance, in case there is a mix-up in the meeting place or time.

If you are giving a presentation, you will probably be asked to provide PowerPoint slides, a hand-out, or electronic file of your poster, in advance of the meeting. Do NOT assume it will be there when you show up: with literally thousands of such files being organized, yours might not be where you want it, when you want it. For slides and videos, bring at least one back-up copy on either a USB pocket drive or DVD—or maybe both. You will have a hard copy of your poster, and some 8.5 x 11 inch reduced copies are also a good idea to hand out in case the meeting organizers don't provide them routinely. Push pin/thumb tacks, an extendable pointer, and perhaps a laser pointer can all come in handy. You may also want to have a paper copy of your slides or poster with you—to review on the plane or during tedious sessions, in advance of your presentation. Check to see if there is a "Speaker-Ready Room" where you can view your slides: you may need to sign in there to confirm your attendance as a presenter as well.

Always acquaint yourself in advance with the audiovisual equipment, microphones, pointers, and layout of any room in which you will give a presentation. Be sure to get to the location of your presentation at least 15 minutes before the entire session starts (not just 15 minutes before you are scheduled to present). Talk to the audiovisual support staff, try the pointers, see how your slides look, assure your cine clips work, etc. Nothing is as disconcerting as starting your talk on pulmonary hemosiderosis just to look up to see prostate cancer slides on the screen.

At the Meeting

Arrive early. Try to arrive before the first session you plan to attend to pick up your registration materials and find your way around. If you are giving a presentation, visit the room or hall where your platform or poster will be presented, and the Speaker Ready Room if one is provided, before the meeting begins.

Wear your name tag. Wear your name tag on your right lapel. This makes it easier to read for those you meet and with whom you shake hands.

Keep your business cards handy. You may meet many new and old colleagues, and exchanging business cards is a way to have up-to-date contact information. Be sure to place the business cards you collect from others in a safe place (wallet or shoulder bag) so you don't lose them on the trip home.

Plan your meals to maximize session attendance. Meals can be difficult. Occasionally, meetings include breakfast, luncheon or dinner, but the majority of the time you are on your own. Concession stands at convention centers can be packed at lunch time—so much so you may choose to skip lunch in order to attend a noon session. Therefore a good breakfast can be most important in sustaining yourself through the long day. Bringing a snack and drink with you can also be a useful option. Vending machines and kiosk vendors may be more accessible than concession stands or on-site restaurants. Occasionally, some convention centers are attached to shopping malls (with food courts) or located close to downtown restaurants. Time is everything here, and you'd hate to miss a valuable presentation because you couldn't get a sandwich in less than 45 minutes.

After You Get Home

You will probably return with a number of acquisitions: notes from sessions you attended, informational material from exhibits and other speakers, business cards from colleagues, and perhaps other documents and materials. Go through them as soon as you return from the meeting, file where appropriate or set aside to be read at a specific time, while your memory of their importance to you is fresh. Too many young physicians end up with piles of paper in their offices or studies, never read or utilized, as they get back into their regular routine. If it was important enough for you to carry it home, it is important enough to address once you get home.

Keep your pocket program with the sessions you attended. You will usually need this to do your on-line evaluations, which are required to secure your CME credit. You can discard it after you have your CME certificate in hand—though occasionally you may need to keep the program, as some organizations require you to document a certain number of topic-specific CME credits (with details of topic, speaker, accrediting body, location and date) to meet criteria to sit for an examination or obtaining a credential. If you are a named speaker listed in the program, definitely keep it as evidence of your accomplishment.

Also, you should be keeping both a CV/portfolio and a CME record. Complete whatever evaluations are required by the meeting sponsors, print your certificate, and record your CME credits and presentation documentation as soon as possible. Don't count on remembering a few days later—you won't.

I always put information from business cards into my electronic phonebook rather than risking losing paper cards. If you do not maintain an electronic phonebook, keep a file specifically for professional contacts so you can find them when needed.

———————◆———————

Large scientific meetings are some of the most enjoyable experiences we have as academic physicians. They enhance your medical knowledge, stimulate thinking outside the box, allow you to interact with professionals from all over the world, and sometimes involve travel to enjoyable locations. An organized approach will assure you maximize your experience—and have fun!

Chapter 13
Notes on Networking

Networking—interacting with other professionals from outside your daily work environment—can be one of the most important activities for successful career development, whether your goal is to grow your practice through increased referrals, find collaborators for innovative research, or gain acknowledgement within your field on a regional, national or international level. To some, networking is easy: they are "naturals" due primarily to their individual personalities and previous social experiences. Others, particularly physicians who have spent long hours studying over the past 10-20 years, are far less comfortable and will need to make more effort to network successfully. Regardless, everyone can improve the productivity and efficiency of their networking efforts.

Goals of Networking
Generally speaking, networking is intended to broaden your professional contacts to include people who can offer more (or different) opportunities than are available from your local working colleagues and staff. Networking goals are specific to your career goals. Practitioners may wish to increase referrals, either generally or for patients with specific conditions or needing particular procedures. Researchers may be seeking collaborators or colleagues to review their work and recommend improvements or new extensions of their investigations. Educators may seek opportunities to participate in national projects, gain membership on important committees, or discover programs others have used to solve challenging educational problems. Administrators may seek advice from other administrators who have faced similar problems of quality, resource utilization, and staffing. Everyone has the chance of learning of new, perhaps better, employment opportunities through networking.

Where to Network?

We all know why Willie Sutton robbed banks. Selecting networking venues is not a dissimilar process. Identifying the types of people you want to meet and with whom to establish relationships is the first step, followed by determining where and how best to meet them. Those seeking patient referrals usually start with county and state medical societies, or offer to provide CME talks at hospitals and practices. Occasionally, tertiary care and clinical research centers, or clinicians seeking distant referrals for unique or experimental treatments, may expand their networking venues to include regional (adjacent counties and states) or national meetings. Researchers typically work in specialized areas with comparatively few colleagues addressing the same or similar scientific questions: for them, national research meetings to present and review posters, platform presentations, and plenary sessions are the place to start—and meetings with more specialization toward their particular research field are always better choices. Clinical investigators may also concentrate on networking with local/regional health care providers to gain referrals of research participants for their clinical trials. Educators may have the broadest selection of opportunities to network, including meetings fully focused on education (AAIM, APDIM, AAMC, etc.) and national medical meetings where some educational issues are presented and discussed. Similarly, administrators have specific organizations (ACPE, IHI, etc.) that sponsor meetings focused on issues of quality, efficiency, regulatory compliance, financing, and related topics. As is the case with medical education programs, national medical organizations are increasingly including administration topics in the programs of their annual meetings.

General Techniques: Pearls, Diamonds and River Rocks

Walking into a large room filled with physicians and other professionals whom you do not know can be awkward, and knowing nothing about those you approach and to whom you introduce yourself can result in very variable returns. The following points are generally applicable to most venues, groups and individuals:

98

Wear a name tag. Place an easily visible name tag on your right upper anterior torso. You will be shaking right hands with people as you meet them, and this makes it easier for them to see your name.

Dress appropriately. Dress like the other attendees dress at the meeting. A Grateful Dead T-shirt and sandals only work at a beach party—and then only if others are sporting similar attire honoring their favorite oldies rock bands as well. Over-dressing is not good either, as a navy suit or formal dress will appear odd when others have selected Dockers, polo shirts and deck shoes to wear to the beach barbecue dinner. When in doubt, the "traditional" academic physician attire is a good choice: for women, a pants suit or slacks with blazer, and low-heel, closed-toe shoes; for men, gray or khaki slacks, neck tie with button-down white or blue shirt, and navy blazer with dark loafers. Your goal should always be to appear to "fit in" rather than "stand out."

Keep your right hand free to shake hands. Keep your right hand clean and dry at receptions, cocktail parties, and other general assemblies. You don't want to need to find a place to put down your crab puffs to be able to shake someone's hand, nor to have cold, wet fingers from your Bud Lite to offer to a new acquaintance.

Be proactive in meeting others. Demonstrate your interest in other attendees first. I have never met a physician without a narcissistic streak, and certainly none who didn't love to talk about themselves. Have a few generic questions ready that can break the ice, and be alert to follow these up with one or two specific questions based on their answers. People are more likely to be amenable to you if you make them feel good, and a new colleague expressing interest in them is a great tool in this regard. In addition, you will find out quickly if this is a person deserving investment of more time and effort on your part, and if they are likely to possess access to the resources you seek.

Keep the walls down. Individuals are very unlikely to approach you if you are with a group of your friends, particularly if it is obvious your group is self-contained or based on previous acquaintances. Also, groups don't approach individuals or smaller groups in these settings.

Try to meet the "big names" in a venue other than a general reception or at one of their presentations. Well-known, senior academicians will be polite but not likely remember you from a busy setting. Committee meetings or membership meetings are better—smaller groups of individuals who already have a common thread based simply on their participation in that group. Some organizations will have "Meet the Leadership" sessions, booths or tables. These are great opportunities to meet prominent scientists and physicians in your field, with the added advantage of your knowing they are there specifically for that reason.

Do your homework. Most major national meetings distribute a program in advance that lists its speakers. Similarly, professional organizations' web sites usually provide public access to membership lists of its committees and work groups. Google and other internet search engines can be invaluable in learning about specific individuals, often including their photographs (though sometimes not recent ones). In addition, such advance research can supply you with conversational topics, perhaps related to their earlier work which you can discuss. A quick search in PubMed or Ovid can also be very useful, particularly if you are relatively new in your field and may not know someone's professional body of work.

Bring business cards. Have business cards easily accessible. Even if you need to go to your local office supply store to get them printed, have several dozen with you at meetings. These should have clear contact information, including telephone and fax numbers, email and mailing address. Don't put your home or cell phone number on these cards, but offer to provide these numbers if you have someone with whom you expect to have ongoing conversations after the meeting ends—this demonstrates your commitment to future communications.

Turn off your cell phone/pager. At a minimum, set them on vibrate only. You WILL be remembered if your communication device disrupts a lecture or meeting, and not in a good way.

Talk with your senior colleagues at your home institution. Not only can they suggest specific individuals to meet, often they can introduce you and help get past the awkwardness of an initial contact.

Try to meet up with past colleagues. Maintain contact with your associates from previous institutions. The wider your networking contacts, the better chance you will have of meeting people who can help you with your career development. A previous professor or program director, a peer from earlier in your training who moved to another school or training program, and even a former trainee can provide a potential avenue to meet the right people.

Relax. Early in your career, your perception of widely known professionals is often idealized. In 30 years or so, you will realize that everyone is pretty much the same: more or less busy perhaps, but we all have families, hobbies, patients—and superiors who cause us grief. Select your comments thoughtfully, but don't anguish over saying "the wrong thing"—well-known, busy academicians will not be keeping a list of people they met whom they didn't like from a brief encounter.

Be positive. Don't be bubbly. Most academic physicians who have been around awhile can identify a disingenuous comment in a New York minute. People enjoy being with others who seem sincere, interested, and congenial, but are suspicious of those who are clearly patronizing, pandering, or "trying too hard."

Be professional. If you are making a presentation at a meeting, know your topic thoroughly. Be able to present without notes, and try not to sound too rehearsed. If you are questioned, answer honestly and thoughtfully—even if you think the interrogator is trying to attack your statements or otherwise confound your presentation. Demonstrating "grace under fire" is a mark of a consummate, confident professional—the kind of person worth knowing (and hiring). During a reception, accept that anyone you meet is of potential value and deserving of a professional greeting and some initial consideration.

After the Meeting
Jot down notes on your way home, while your memory is fresh. Always follow-up with an email or phone call if you promised to do so, but give it a few days to allow your new contacts to get home and catch up after a busy meeting, and so you don't appear too anxious. If new colleagues said they would contact you, it is probably best to give them two weeks or so before initiating contact yourself. Everyone has their own individual definitions of timelines, but sometimes people do forget and may thank you for reminding them.

———————◆———————

Networking is an art. We live in an era of constant review and improvement—in practice, education and administration. Networking is no different. Pay attention to what works for you, and what doesn't work so well. Observe others, talk to your peers and mentors. Polish your skills. With time, networking can become comfortable and natural even for the most introverted among us. Don't expect perfection at first, or perhaps ever. But directed effort at improving your networking skills will be time well spent over the course of your career.

Chapter 14
Notes on Manuscript Reviewing

Almost all academic physicians and other scientists volunteer their time to review manuscripts submitted for peer-reviewed (refereed) publication. Doing so establishes a "national reputation" required for promotion and/or tenure, enhances your contributions to your fields of expertise, and is the first step toward membership on editorial boards and associate editor appointments. In addition, this process will strengthen your critical reading abilities as you become a better consumer of professional literature, and will often enhance your own writing skills. A few journals will award you CME credit for the reviews you perform, but this practice is unusual.

Selecting Journals for Manuscript Review
Since peer-reviewed journals receive a large number of submitted manuscripts, most journals are always looking for scholars to serve as reviewers. Many journals will ask you to review if they publish an article you have authored. The most elite journals are highly selective in selecting their reviewers, but most others will have you review one or two manuscripts in order to judge your abilities as a reviewer when you first volunteer. When starting out, pick low- to mid-level journals (impact factors of, say, between 1 and 3). Start with the journals you read on a regular basis, which publish on topics with which you are familiar and generally up-to-date. A journal where physicians such as you are the target audience is your best bet.

Volunteering your Reviewer Services
You should send an email or letter, along with your CV, to the editorial office of the journal(s) you have selected, volunteering your services as an ad hoc reviewer. Introduce yourself, including your academic rank, school, hospital, and type of practice (e.g., hospitalist, ambulatory care, subspecialist, etc.) and how long you have been practicing; compliment the journal and convey that you read it regularly; and

note that you have the time, interest, and desire to contribute as a reviewer. If you are just starting out, you may want to ask a senior faculty member to help you with your first few reviews—and include this fact in your letter. Identify two or three topical areas of expertise in which you are willing to review; these should be areas relevant to your practice and teaching, where you are comfortable with your knowledge of the latest applicable science, so you will not need to perform extensive background reading to provide a quality review. They should be fairly specific: "antihypertensive pharmacology" rather than "cardiology"; "pathophysiology of diabetic nephropathy" rather than "diabetic complications." Also, if you already review for one or more journals, including this fact in your letter will convey your experience as an established peer reviewer.

You can usually expect to hear back in a month or so from the editor confirming your inclusion in the reviewer pool for the journal. At that time, visit the journal web site (virtually all reviews are now submitted electronically) and become familiar with its format (most have a word limit, separate comments for authors and editor, and often recommended issues to be addressed in the comments—such as relevance, validity of methods, appropriateness of conclusions, limitations, etc.). In addition to your written comments, most journals will ask you to grade the paper on specific areas (e.g., 1-5 scores on a half dozen questions) and perhaps give an overall priority score (0-100) on the paper's value and importance. Though you will usually be asked for a specific recommendation (e.g., "Accept," "Accept with minor revisions," "Accept with major revisions," "Reject with comments," "Reject"), you should not state your recommendation in the comments viewed by the authors; that decision is up to the editor, who may or may not agree with your assessment.

Role and Process: Practical Points
One of the most crucial issues to editors is assuring reviews are completed and returned promptly. The time you have to review a manuscript is generally between one and three weeks, and the time window has been shrinking as journals

seek to get an answer to authors as soon as possible. AL-
WAYS GET YOUR REVIEWS SUBMITTED BY THE
DEADLINE!! Missing your deadline will guarantee you won't
be asked to review again for that journal.

When you receive an invitation, it is acceptable to occasionally turn it down—do so when your available time is very
limited (e.g., traveling, on service, on vacation); when the
topic is way outside your area of expertise; or the study type
(e.g., lab science, epidemiology) is outside your scope of
practice. Don't do this too often, however; you may not be
asked to review again if you turn down several sequential
invitations.

Ad hoc reviewers briefly summarize manuscripts, provide an opinion based on their analysis, identify strengths
and weakness in the work, suggest changes to strengthen
the paper whenever possible, and make a recommendation
to the editor. No manuscript will be accepted or rejected
solely on your recommendation—at least two, and often
three or more reviewers will assess each submission, and
the editorial board member will adjudicate discrepancies and
make a final decision.

No one is an expert on everything, even within a narrow
discipline. As such, you may want to recommend additional
reviews, such as a separate statistical review on complex
meta-analyses or database studies. Even when you cannot
comment on the entire article, your comments are still of
value to the journal—this should not lead you to turn down
reviews *per se*.

Your role is as a professional/scientist, NOT a high
school English teacher! Do not waste time and space cor-
recting grammar, spelling and punctuation—journals employ
literary editorial assistants, who are usually far better at this
than are most physicians. Conversely, if you feel the paper
is poorly written, difficult to read, or the overall writing is below the standard of the journal, be sure to say so in the
comments to the editor.

Finally, a note on confidentiality. Usually you are asked
to sign a confidentiality agreement when you first begin to
review for a journal. Even if not, it is assumed that you will
not disclose any information from the paper until it is pub-

lished, and not disclose any information whatsoever if it is rejected. If accepted, the paper belongs to the journal, not the reviewers. Once the review process for a given paper is complete, you must destroy any and all copies you have of the manuscript (paper or electronic). You should keep a copy of your review until the final decision is made, however; though many journals will send you a copy of your comments if a revision is submitted (see below), some do not and having this copy will save you time later.

Performing a Manuscript Review

You should probably commit a half day (four-to-five hours) each to your first few reviews. Eventually you will become more efficient, and one-to-two hours is average for an experienced reviewer. You may need to read some of the references, or check other literature, before completing the review.

Everyone develops his or her own approach to reviewing, as will you with time and experience. The following is a generic approach that works well for many people, and is a good way to start your reviewing.

1. Read the article as a consumer. Just read it—don't analyze, write comments, etc. Read it as you would a published article in that journal. If you feel you have a reasonable understanding of the article from a single reading that is a positive sign. If not....

2. Read it a second time, highlighting or writing notes on key issues. What isn't clear or doesn't make sense? Does the article assume common knowledge that is not known to you? Are there any obvious issues that could affect the validity of the study or applicability of the results to the general population? Did you note anything novel or innovative?

3. From your notes and highlights, make a brief outline of the article. The reviewer site may suggest a specific outline format, or you may develop your own to use regularly. An outline assures you have identified and consid-

ered the key aspects of the paper. A reasonable outline addresses the following questions:

A. *Is the topic important?*
   Clinical care, scientific understanding, public health, economics, policy, etc.

B. *What is the purpose of the article?*
   1. Answer a question
   2. Report a new or unusual observation
   3. Summarize present knowledge
   4. Present and support an opinion
   5. Identify needs (research, funding, policy, etc.)
   6. Other

C. *What type of article is it?*
   1. Original clinical research
      a. Meta-analysis
      b. Randomized clinical trial
      c. Observational study
         i. Prospective cohort
         ii. Case-control
         iii. Cross-sectional
      d. Retrospective
         i. Database/registry
         ii. Post-hoc analysis
         iii. Epidemiology, historical
   2. Review
      a. Systematic or quantitative (formal search, article inclusion/exclusion criteria)
      b. Narrative or qualitative
      c. Clinical update
   3. Report
      a. Case series
      b. Case report
   4. Opinion
      a. Editorial
      b. Commentary
      c. Position/Consensus Statement

D. *Are the methods appropriate and valid?* (This is a separate and quite extensive topic beyond the scope of this chapter.)

E. *Are the results plausible?*
   1. Are they consistent with other work in the area, or are differences explicable for logical reasons?
   2. Do they fit with clinical observations, related research, or established epidemiology?

F. *Are the conclusions supported?*
   1. Do they follow from the findings?
   2. Any major flaws in reasoning?
   3. Strength of conclusions appropriate?
      a. Association
      b. Causality
      c. Parallel but unrelated
   4. Clinical vs. statistical significance?

G. *Are potential applications of the conclusions important?*
   1. Author's opinion
   2. Your opinion

H. *What are the authors' statement of limitations regarding the study/work?*

You should comment separately on tables and figures. These are costly to publish, and should enhance and clarify the information, rather than repeating information from the text. For most articles, information from the text should not be repeated in tables. Some tables and figures add little to the work, and you may recommend some be removed or consolidated. Sometimes additional information is needed in a table (p values, for example), and this should also be recommended if needed.

Writing your Comments
Until you are very facile at both reviewing and using the specific reviewer web site for your journal, it is prudent to

write your comments on a separate word processor document, then cut and paste them into the reviewer site. Be sure to spell check and proof read your work—it never looks good if your comments need editing.

Comments to authors. You first should summarize the paper in two or three sentences. Second, address methods and point out strengths and weaknesses; include comments on appropriateness of the statistical tests used, sources of bias, study size and duration, and any other factors you deem important. Third, review the results presented, including significance, plausibility, and consistency with other studies. Fourth, address the authors' conclusions in interpreting their results. Fifth, address the stated potential application of their data to the health care field. Limitations of the work can be addressed in each section or summarized separately at the end. Finally, make specific recommendations on changes you feel would make the paper better—clearer, more accurate, more readable, more concise—i.e., more publishable.

Try to sound positive, even if the article is terrible—remember your own experiences as an author. Few papers are all bad or all good. Regardless of your opinion of the article, the authors put considerable time and work into their manuscript, and they deserve to be respected for the effort.

Comments to the editor. If asked to submit separate comments to the editor *that the authors will not see*, make them brief and do not repeat information from your author-directed comments. These might include whether the topic or type of article is appropriate for this journal and its target readership; whether you think there is useful information present but the article as written is simply not publishable; whether a formal literary editorial review, or statistical review, is needed; or if, after several readings, you still have no idea what the authors were trying to say. The strength of your opinions can be included here.

Numerical grading. Many journals will ask you to assign a number grade for various aspects of the paper. These might include applicability to the readership of the journal, clinical relevance, quality of the science, readability of the paper, and other assessments. There is no "gold standard" here, so think about the published articles you have read over your career for comparison. As you continue to review for a given journal, you will begin to standardize these grades in your own mind. As a check, when you hear back on the final decision, see how often the editor's opinion concurs with yours and yours with that of the other reviewers.

Follow-up, feedback and revisions. You can expect to receive a thank you letter or email from the editor for your service. You should print and save this for your portfolio as documentation of your scholarly work. Also, keep a copy of your review. Most journals will notify you, usually by email, of the final decision. Most journals also give you access to the other reviewers' comments—which can be a great learning experience for you.

Reviewing a revised manuscript. Opinions differ here, but I recommend you always agree to review the revised manuscript if the authors choose to submit one. You have already spent time analyzing the paper, so even major revisions should be easily checked against your original comments. This is an important service to the journal. Most authors will submit a letter along with their revision, and should address each comment/recommendation made in the review. In addition to confirming that necessary changes have been made, assure the revision is readable, clear, and appropriate for publication on this second review. If the revision still leaves the manuscript unacceptable, don't be afraid to say so; some authors can be so arrogant as to discard your recommendations—they should be sending their work somewhere else.

Accompanying editorials. Often reviewers are asked if an editorial should accompany the paper if it is published. Normally, major clinical studies, important new findings, novel treatment paradigms, and reports that suggest a change in physician thinking, diagnostics or risk assessment can be enhanced by a thoughtful editorial. An editorial can also place the paper in perspective, in light of other reports on the topic. You can recommend an editorial be performed even if you do not feel qualified to write one yourself; conversely, if you are confident in the breadth and depth of your knowledge of the field, you may choose to offer to write the editorial if the editor deems appropriate.

————————◆————————

Good editors understand that your time is valuable and will usually request four or fewer reviews from you each year (unless you take a special assignment through an affiliated professional organization, or become a member of the editorial board). However, with the facility of electronic communication technology, a few journals have chosen to send review requests automatically on every manuscript submitted on reviewers' topic areas; these editors expect you to read every abstract as soon as you receive it and accept or refuse each request, and if it takes a day or two, you might do the initial screening only to discover the journal has already assigned the reviews to others. In my opinion, this is an abuse of the relationship and you should seriously consider removing your name from the reviewer pools of these journals. You receive no credit, and provide no useful service to the scientific community, through this time-consuming process. There are plenty of valuable, high-quality publications needing reviewers, with editors who appreciate how valuable your donated time is to you—and to them.

That being said, no good deed ever goes unpunished. The better job you do, the more reviewer invitations you can expect to receive. If you feel you are being asked to provide more service than you have time to contribute, contact the editor and ask that you receive a smaller number of invitations. For your own career development, it is better to review four articles per year for three different journals than one each month for a single journal, especially during your first few years as a reviewer. Your editorial experience will broaden by working with different types of publications and different editors, and add to your resume accordingly.

Also, no relationship is interminable. Although a few academicians do review for some journals for twenty or more years, it is very reasonable to resign from the ad hoc reviewer pool after several years as you add more prestigious journals to your reviewing experience, or when your career re-directs to different specific disciplines. Doing so also "makes room" for younger physicians to take your place as you grow to review for international, signature publications within your field.

Chapter 15
Notes on Medical Writing
(for the Beginning Author)

Below are some general suggestions that will help you get through the various steps of scientific/professional publication. Though not exhaustive, following these recommendations will permit for fewer rewrites, better time utilization (for you and your senior author) and hasten the point when you can write without a senior mentor (or become one yourself).

Selecting a Preferred Journal
It is a very good idea to select a preferred journal before you start writing; when possible, you should email the editorial office to be sure the journal will consider the type of article, as well as its topic, you plan to submit. By looking through earlier issues of the journal and its "Instructions to Authors," you will have a good sense of whether it will consider the type of article you plan to write. However, some journals have a one-year backlog of accepted papers and, if your topic is similar to those already in its queue, it may be rejected simply to avoid duplication. One note: most journals no longer publish simple case reports, and fewer will publish narrative (qualitative) review articles unless they are invited manuscripts.

Also, each journal has a "profile" (expertise level) of its target readership; don't plan to submit an article to a primary care journal if only PhD psychopharmacologists are likely to understand it. Be realistic, but not timid—better to shoot too high and resubmit later than shoot too low and never get published in better journals.

Another good idea is to make sure there isn't a similar or (worse) definitive article recently published. You won't be adding anything of value to the literature. Editors read other journals, so they will know.

Spend a few hours in the library or on-line, do some brief searches, and speak to senior faculty active in the field. Forethought and background work are both good time investments.

Outline

Your outline should be no more than 1-1½ pages in length and should NOT be exhaustive; it is a way to organize your ideas, arrange them logically, and make appropriate subordinate subtopics so the presentation makes sense. Use outlining functions or indentations. Use phrases, not sentences. Brief is best.

Organization equals clarity. A well-organized article helps the reader understand what you are saying and where each idea fits into the overall topic. Like a good lecture, the organization of the materials in your paper should stand out, and an initial outline helps you achieve this.

Outlines also help you keep "apples with apples and oranges with oranges"; e.g., if you are going to have three tests to confirm a diagnosis and four different treatments (each with specific patient types, contra-indications, doses, and recommended follow-up), the outline allows you to visualize this up front and write to the outline: the two major subheadings are "Diagnosis" and "Treatment." Within the first major subheading, "Diagnosis," you would include three subordinate subheadings: one for each of the three tests you will be describing. Within the second major subheading, "Treatment," you would include four subordinate subheadings: one for each of the different treatments. Moreover, you would want to describe each of the treatments in a roughly equal fashion; for example, you wouldn't want to allocate two paragraphs to describing the first treatment, one paragraph to describing the second treatment, and one sentence to describing each of the third and fourth treatments, if they are roughly equivalent considerations.

Outlining also helps you with rewrites. If you end up way over your word limit, you can go back to your outline to help you symmetrically reduce volume among all components of a subheading equally; for example, reducing the description of each of your four treatments from four paragraphs to four sentences.

First Draft

When writing an initial draft to be reviewed by your senior author, try to have your manuscript approximate the maximum word count for the selected journal and article type. It is difficult to reduce a 5,000 word manuscript to 1,750 words after it's all done!

I always recommend writing the Introduction and Summary/Conclusion last. Once you have a good idea of how the body of your article will read, you can make the Introduction more succinct and the Summary/Conclusion parallel the organization of your text.

An introduction should be brief: establish the importance of the topic ("CHF affects 1.2 million Americans annually") and the question you are trying to address in your article ("Published guidelines fail to identify preferred treatment options for specific patient subpopulations with concurrent diseases"). You don't need the history of the disease—doctors usually know CHF is generally bad and living longer is generally good. . . .

1. Use an 11 or 12 point san serif font such as Arial. Double space and leave one-inch margins all around.
2. Number the pages, including the title page.
3. Place sections in the following order on a *single* word processing document for your first draft:
   A. Title Page
   B. Abstract
   C. Body (text)
   D. References
   E. Tables in order
   F. Figures in order
   G. Figure legends
4. Run spelling and grammar checks.

Define all abbreviations the first time they are mentioned. This must be done separately in the abstract, text, and in the legend of each figure or table. Use abbreviations sparingly as they make the paper harder to read. Very common, standard abbreviations are usually OK once defined (CHF, MI, CKD). If you have one or two terms that you use repeatedly, it is usually worthwhile to make an abbreviation with first use, then use the abbreviation throughout the text, as this will reduce word count significantly: e.g., PE for pulmonary embolus, VTE for venous thromboembolic disease, RA for rheumatoid arthritis, etc. Never use slang or common terms—you are writing for a professional journal, not Facebook.

Use standard units for any values given: mg/dL, IU/hr, etc. Most U.S. journals allow English units, but a few require SI or both. Such abbreviations ARE standard and do not need to be defined in the text.

Use original tables when doing so will help you either present the information more clearly or cut the word count in the text. *Do NOT repeat* information in a table AND text; this only lengthens the paper unnecessarily and will materially decrease your chance for publication.

Although copyright-protected tables and figures can be included (you must obtain legal release for their re-publication), it is far better to create your own. This eliminates the release process (which can delay publication), and is more likely to give you products that more closely support your article.

Be consistent in your stylistic choices. For example, if expressing concentrations in mEq/L, use these units for all similar concentrations, rather than switching between mmol/L, mg/dL, etc.

If inserting references at this time, do not number them as they may be moved around. Use first author last name, journal and year in text (Jones, Am J Med 2010). If you have two or more articles where all this is the same, add the first page after the year to differentiate. If you anticipate multiple drafts, it is sometimes better just to mark where a supporting reference will be entered, and insert the actual reference when you are closer to a final version.

Never start a sentence with an Arabic numeral or abbreviation. Use "Twenty-seven" instead of "27," "Angiotensin converting enzyme inhibitor" instead of "ACE inhibitor," etc. at the beginning of a sentence.

Enter your full bibliographic references after the text so an accurate estimate of word count can be made. Use the standard NLM format. Include *all* authors (don't use *et al.* at this time as journals vary in their requirements), Volume and Issue, and full first and last page (e.g., 1145-1148; *not* 1145-

48). Note that authors are listed as last name, space, first (and middle) initials without separating punctuation. With the title, capitalize only the first letter of the first word, the first letter of a word following a colon, and proper names. No spaces are to be included between year, volume, issue, and pages (spaces are unnecessary and add to automated word counts). Use official journal abbreviations as found in Pub-Med/NLM:

Jones AB, Smith CD, Brown TC, Gray L. This is how to write an article: Do it right the first time Mr. Doctor. *Am J Med.* 2008;21(6):1145-1148.

Later Drafts

Use as few words as possible. Write concisely and make every word count. Length adds to the cost of publishing your article, and therefore reduces the chance it will be published. Avoid phrases that only add length and no content: "It has been said that CHF kills people (ref)" vs. "CHF kills people (ref)." For most articles, phrases such as "According to Smith et al., ... (ref) are unnecessary; if you are citing the reference, readers will see it is Dr. Smith's article you are citing. Also, stay away from passive tense, which adds up to 10-15 percent to your text length—people think it makes papers sound more formal, but it doesn't. Use present rather than past tense when possible, as this will also allow you to use fewer words.

Other tricks to reduce length: use adjective forms instead of predicates: "RA complications" instead of "complications of RA"; "accepted PE therapy" instead of "accepted therapy for PE."

Avoid repeating terms over and over, particularly technical or lengthy terms close together in the text. Try to find synonyms, use pronouns, or combine simple sentences into complex sentences with a single subject. Don't be afraid to use a dictionary or thesaurus. They are still popular books for a reason.

Stay away from personal references as much as possible. "We think" or "I recommend" or "we support the approach" shouldn't be used; simply stated, nobody cares what we think or what you recommend. It is what the *evidence* supports and what the *literature* recommends that matters.

Minimize your use of font modifiers. Too many bold, underlined, capitalized or italicized words make a paper look cheap, like you are writing an advertisement for a new hair restoration product. Use these for very specific reasons (e.g., similar subtopic titles all in bold; subtopics within a paragraph underlined) to make the organization of the paper clearer.

Final Draft

Read and follow the journal's "Instructions to Authors" *carefully* and *completely*. Print out a copy and check off each instruction when completed, as if you were preparing your income tax forms (both are written at a 4th grade level). There is no excuse for not doing this. Ignoring instructions aggravates the editor, the reviewer and the editorial staffers—and suggests disrespect for their journal.

Pay particular attention to statements regarding conflict of interest, authorship qualification and involvement in the manuscript preparation, copyright release, IRB approval, funding and support, etc. as often a journal will not even review your manuscript until these issues are addressed as instructed. Each journal has different requirements—some want this information on the title page, some in a cover letter, and some in a series of separate documents. Do *exactly* as instructed.

Comply with how the journal wants its submissions organized. Some journals want a single document; some want a separate abstract, or a separate AND included abstract; some want tables separate, some table/figure legends separate, some with all figure legends on one page, etc.

Note not only the journal's limit on word count but also how word counts are defined by the specific journal. Sometimes it is a total word count, including figures, title page, etc. Sometimes, particularly when that journal requires additional information on the title page, the title page is excluded from the count. Other times, references may be excluded, or tables/figures excluded. Although word counts are rarely absolute (i.e., a few words over will not cause an otherwise acceptable article to be rejected), if you miss how they count words you may think you are under the limit but in fact be way over.

Pay attention to the total number of tables and figures that the journal will accept for each of its articles—which is as important as total word count. If it is absolutely essential that you include an extra table or figure beyond the stated limit, email the editorial office before submitting the manuscript and ask permission. If granted, state in your cover letter that you received this permission.

Always include a list of "Key Words" (3-5 MeSH terms), a running title (brief title to be placed atop each page), a clinical significance statement, and anything else that the specific journal requires.

If you think you are done with your final draft, put the paper away for a few days and come back and read it as if it were a new article. You will be amazed at the number of changes that should be made that you did not notice when you were immersed in the writing. Time permitting, have others—friends, colleagues, relatives, intelligent pets—read it and give you feedback.

Issues Specific to Research Articles, Meta-analyses, and Systematic Reviews

Your Introduction should clearly state your hypothesis or the specific aim(s) of your study.

Your Methods section is crucial. It should be sufficiently detailed for the readers to be able to reproduce your study (along with the references in this section). In general, it is better to over-write than under-write experimental methods—these can always be cut down later. Clearly define your dependent variable(s) (endpoint, outcome) stating which is primary (i.e., used in the power analysis), which is/are secondary, etc. Clearly define your independent variables and explain why you are handling them the way you are. Include brand names and the company used for assays, statistical programs/versions used for analysis, how variables were measured, how participants were selected for the study (sequential, inclusion/exclusion criteria, etc.), how medical records were reviewed and who reviewed them. Make sure you understand why individual statistical tests were used, and of course that you used the right ones—many manuscripts have been rejected because the investigators used tests that made their data look good, but were totally inappropriate for the data collected, or when their study violated the assumptions of individual tests, making the significance statements of the results invalid.

Systematic reviews should clearly state the search engine (PubMed, Ovid, etc.) and version or date used, search terms that were included, time span of articles included in your review, exclusion criteria (size, insufficient detail in paper, review rather than original research article, etc.); whether you used secondary references (i.e., articles referenced in those you found in your search) and your criteria for using them. The key to a systematic review is to have a pre-defined system to identify and include/exclude published articles and then to stick to that system—don't be arbitrary. Also, defining outcomes (included papers) for a systematic review is also crucial—you cannot compare studies that only measured symptom improvement with those showing hard mortality benefits. The Results section is for results—not your interpretation of the results. Do not interject commentary, explanations, or other qualifying verbiage in the Results section. Save this for the Discussion section, or at most make a short reference that it will be addressed later in the article: *"One study[3] did not find an effect, but this may have been due to a pre-selected study population (see Discussion)."*

The Results section in a systematic review often must be organized after the data are collected—in other words, the data drives the organization of the results that you may not know prior to your search. For example, in doing a systematic review of treatments for heart failure, you may not anticipate there would be a wealth of literature on chronic intermittent CVVH until you do the search; therefore you will need a section of your results on this treatment, whether or not you anticipated finding it.

The Results section for a clinical trial should start with a population description, by category if appropriate. Make sure you emphasize that groups (treatment, control) were similar in all major categories that could potentially affect the results, and if not say so clearly and deal with it in the Discussion. Random selection takes care of a lot of chance bias if, in fact, random selection occurred.

The Discussion section is the most variable in length, content, and intent. Some will present great detail of previously-published studies or reviews, contrasting your manuscript/study to earlier works. Others may summarize accepted knowledge and practice in the field, and then point out how the new information in this paper adds to or modifies that body of information. Every Discussion section should, first, clearly state the findings of the paper. Also, every paper presenting new data or having identified literature in a systematic way should always include one paragraph describing the limitations of your study. No study is perfect, and most are not completely bad—99 percent are somewhere in between; if YOU list your limitations and how they may have influenced your findings, the reviewers won't think they found something major that you missed—and therefore suspect there are additional flaws in your paper. The remainder of this section, however, should be driven by available remaining length and your intent for a "take home message" from the paper.

Submitting Your Manuscript
Almost all journals take submissions on-line; these systems walk you through the submission but you MUST follow the instructions. Be sure to write down the account name, password, and manuscript number given to you so you can track/refer to the article during future communications and to enter revisions.

You should hear something back in eight weeks or so. If not, you should inquire as to the status of your paper. Sometimes you can do this by checking the submission website using your assigned tracking number; other times an email to the editorial office is best.

Revisions. It is very unusual to have a manuscript accepted without revision on the initial submission. Most will require at least "minor revisions," which might include changing a few sentences, omitting a table or figure, removing home-made abbreviations, or softening a statement in the conclusions. Most of the time, it is best to just make these changes and resubmit promptly. As long as the content and meaning is not materially changed, these are battles best left un-fought. Also, many times the reviewers are extremely knowledgeable about your paper's topic, and their recommendations will improve the paper. Revisions should be accompanied by a cover letter thanking the reviewers for their comments, addressing every recommendation by each reviewer and clearly stating the changes that have been made, and, finally, stating you believe their suggestions have made the paper stronger (whether you believe it or not).

Sometimes there will be lots of recommended revisions. You may find most of the recommended revisions acceptable but strongly oppose a small number of the revisions being proposed. In these circumstances, begin your letter with a summary of all the changes you DID make. Then craft a detailed, well-referenced argument for the one or two recommended revisions you did NOT make, and why you feel those shouldn't be made. Don't be afraid to pile on the evidence supporting your decision not to make a change—most reviewers are unpaid, busy, and will cave under sufficient pressure of having to rebut your 78-point defense.

Sometimes the reviewers are inappropriate and want so many things changed you would have to rewrite the entire article; they may simply not like the topic, or your affiliation, or have pre-conceived notions on who should be "allowed" to write on the topic you have chosen—reviewing is a very subjective process. You should discuss a strategy with your senior author before considering a major re-write, but usually submission to another journal is appropriate in this type of instance.

Pay attention to time lines. Normally the reviews will be accompanied by a letter from the editor saying they will re-review/reconsider if the changes are addressed, and they will give you a reasonable timeline. You MUST have your revised manuscript submitted by this time or they may not re-review it.

Acceptance. Your work isn't over once the manuscript is accepted. You can expect several additional communications from the journal prior to publication: these are almost always by email. Copyright release statements and conflict of interest forms (often signed by each contributing author), institutional releases, and other legal paperwork must precede actual publication. Do these promptly—faster is better.

A month or more before the publication date, you will receive the "galley proof." This will look like your article printed as the journal will print it, with headings, formatting, and other details. Many journals now are automatically having literary editing done by their staff, which may be reflected only in the galleys. You may be surprised at how little time they give you to review the galleys—often as little as 48 hours. However, that should be plenty—don't feel pressured; just accept it as standard operating procedure. All you need do is read the article and make sure everything says what it should say. Do NOT get into stylistic issues here—that stage is long past. All you want to do is make sure the literary/grammar changes, additions and deletions did not change the meaning of any statements. If changes are needed, I suggest you BOTH make pen-and-ink changes on a hard copy (faxed back to the publisher) or use the on-line editor functions provided by the journal web site (if available), AND return/include a descriptive email or letter with the changes listed (e.g., page 2, para 2, line 3: change "vagrancies" to "vagaries"). This is the best way to assure the final published product says what you want.

Finally, in this day of electronic media, purchasing reprints is just dumb. They are very expensive to buy, need to be stored, and are expensive to mail should you get reprint requests from outside. A pdf file is ideal, and if the publisher won't provide you with one, it is worth having your librarian get one for you (even if you have to pay the typical $15 fee for it). You can then keep it on a CD or hard drive, email it all over the world for free, and print a fresh hard copy of your article whenever needed.

Rejections. Don't be too disappointed if your article is rejected. There are lots of reasons this happens, many of which do not mean you wrote a bad article. Inappropriate readership audience, a particularly malignant reviewer (sometimes with their own political or ego-centric agenda), recently published similar article, too complex for readership—these and other reasons can lead a journal to reject your well-written manuscript.

Read the reviewer comments (if provided) objectively. They are rejecting a written paper, not your personal or spiritual value on the planet. Often their ideas are sound and you can re-write your article using them and have a better chance of acceptance on subsequent submissions to another journal. Discuss these with your senior author.

Lessons Learned

Like most things in life, you will get better at scientific writing with each experience—including the lessons learned from manuscripts that were never accepted for publication. Smart people make mistakes—just not the same one twice. Early in your writing career, start a notebook of big and little things you learned with each article you wrote, and make sure your next article corrects/addresses the issues you previously encountered. You will improve faster with this process, and you will have some notes from which you can write tutorials for your future junior colleagues (like the one you are reading now).

———————◆———————

Remember, we all went into medicine to help people have better lives. Scientific writing is an impact multiplier toward that goal. Rather than helping 50 patients, your 50 hours of writing work will translate into hundreds, perhaps thousands, of other health care providers using your article to help their patients, over and over during their professional careers. Choose to make a bigger impact, to help more patients in more ways and more places than you could possibly do otherwise, and you will find it is well worth the effort.

And have fun! My first paper took six months, more than 20 rewrites, and so much red ink from my mentor that he made me buy him a box of red pens for my second paper. I considered a career change to either animal husbandry or accounting. Now, more than a quarter century later, I find writing with junior colleagues among my favorite activities, and experience great joy in their successful publication. If you make the commitment, there is no reason you cannot experience the same satisfaction and make the same kind of impact. There are few "natural" writers, just as there are few natural teachers, or clinicians, or musicians. It takes dedicated work to become proficient. You *will* succeed if you *choose* to succeed.

Chapter 16
Notes on Writing an Abstract

An abstract is a brief summary of a larger work. Abstracts serve as introductory summaries of larger papers, typically research or case reports, and are usually available through literature search engines to the academic community. They also are used in the competitive process of selecting submissions for platform or poster presentations at professional meetings and local or regional symposia. Specifics of formatting are dictated by the journal or organization sponsoring the meeting. However, abstracts have many things in common, and the ability to prepare a well-written, competitive abstract is an absolute must for academic physicians.

Some Common Facts about Abstracts

1. They must be able to stand alone. Whether introducing a full manuscript or posted as part of a presentation, an abstract must be able to be read and fully understood without reference to any other materials.

2. Every organization and journal has very specific formatting requirements for abstracts. These include word count, font type and size, use of capitals or font modifiers, how authors and affiliated institutions are listed, whether tables or graphs are permitted, acceptable word processing programs/file types, and whether a structured or unstructured format (see below) should be used. It is essential that the formatting requirements be followed carefully to avoid having your abstract disqualified from further consideration just because it is formatted incorrectly.

3. Brevity is KEY. The most difficult skill for most authors is meeting the word count/space limitations. A concise writing style is essential—avoid all unnecessary words, passive tense, hedging qualifiers, and excessive detail. You will inevitably want to include more information than

there is space to accommodate, so pick your facts and words carefully. Leave out useless statements such as "More research is needed"—more research is ALWAYS needed, and the reader will not find such statements of value. However, limit use of abbreviations, especially non-standard ones; these make reading difficult and could adversely affect your score on competitive grading. Include only the most essential information—if successful, you will have ample opportunity to add detail in your complete manuscript, or during your platform or poster presentation.

4. Know your audience and reviewers. A highly specialized journal or organization is likely to have reviewers very familiar with your research techniques and areas; hence background information can be brief. General medical meetings may have comparatively few reviewers, who likely know far less about your specific field; they will require less technical information but more detail on the potential impact of your work. *Write for the people reading your abstract.*

5. Make it clear and easy to read. A reviewer may be comparing 50-100 or more abstracts assigned to them. Those that are difficult to read, require repeated readings to understand, or provide information without obvious relation to the topic will usually be graded lower, even if the research itself was superior. Use standard formal English grammar, and check your spelling and punctuation.

6. In general, even if they are permitted, try to avoid figures and graphs unless they are essential to conveying your concepts or results. Graphics take up significant space and limit your available text so severely that they often have a net negative effect on the impact of the abstract. This is not always the case but if considering a graph or table, get some additional opinions from colleagues or mentors before including them (see below).

7. Be sure to limit numerical data to significant figures only. More decimal places do NOT necessarily make your results more exact—but they do suggest you might be unfamiliar with some elementary research and reporting principles.

8. Other basic concepts of scientific writing apply to abstracts as well. Make sure your work is complete before writing the abstract. Finish writing well before the submission deadline, put it on the shelf for a few days, and re-read what you wrote (you may be surprised by the result!). Ask colleagues, both within your field and from other disciplines, to critique your abstract early enough so you can consider their suggested changes; colleagues from outside the field may in fact offer the most useful comments, as they may be more representative of reviewers at a large/general professional meeting or broad-scope journal. I usually set a "drop dead" date at least 48 hours before the submission deadline. If electronic submission is not an option, this personal deadline should be at least 72 hours.

Structured vs. Unstructured Abstracts
Abstracts are classified as "structured" or "unstructured" but a better terminology would be "labeled" or "unlabeled," since the organization and information are basically the same for both categories. A structured abstract includes formal subheadings, such as *Title*, *Authors and Affiliations*, followed by the body—typically composed of *Introduction* or *Background*, *Objective* (which may be included alternatively in the Introduction), *Methods*, *Results*, and *Conclusions* (and perhaps *Significance of Findings* or *Clinical Applicability*). An unstructured abstract usually has the same material in the same sequence, but subheading titles are excluded by formatting requirements. Therefore, aside from section headings, preparing either a structured or unstructured abstract requires a similar process.

Components of an Abstract

(The *Title, Authors and Affiliated Institution discussion applies only to abstracts submitted for platform or poster presentation**; manuscript abstracts usually do not include these as separate listings within the abstract. Although section headings are used below for structured abstracts, these same sections are included, but without the section titles, in unstructured abstracts.)

Title.* Papers selected for poster or platform presentation will be listed by the title you submit on the abstract. There are always letter limitations to avoid large variations in title length among selected papers. Meeting attendees will decide on whether to come to your presentation based on the title, and those wandering the large poster halls will be attracted (or not) by your title. Titles should be concise but descriptive, reflecting the few critical aspects of your presentation. They should be neither too broad nor too narrow: "Tumor necrosis factor activates leukocytes in a porcine model of pulmonary hypertension" is preferable to either "Tumor necrosis factor activates superoxide anion formation resulting in elevated arteriolar resistance in a porcine model of pulmonary hypertension" or "Tumor necrosis factor causes pulmonary hypertension." Titles should never have non-standard abbreviations, nor introduce abbreviations for the rest of the abstract.

Authors.* Names must be formatted according to the abstract instructions. Just as in a manuscript, first author is *Lead*, last author is *Senior*, others are *Contributing*. You will usually be asked to confirm that all listed individuals meet criteria for authorship (e.g., ACP, AMA, or society/journal definitions), any real or apparent conflicts of interest are fully disclosed, all funding sources for your work are reported, and the research being presented was performed according to ethical guidelines and with the approval of your Institutional Review Board (human research) and/or IACUC (animal research) (or similar oversight body). You may in fact be required to sign a written statement to these effects, and perhaps even have all your co-authors do likewise. Allow time for this.

Affiliated Institutions.* List only the institution of the lead author on the abstract unless instructions specifically stipulate otherwise; for a five-author abstract with each author being from a different institution, affiliation listings could consume half your writing space. Again, follow directions given by the sponsoring organization or journal, and don't include more information than is required (e.g., zip codes or street addresses may not be needed). Be sure, however, that when you are presenting your work the poster or title slide includes all authors' affiliations.

Body. Once you have the obligate information of title, authors and affiliated institutions, work within the remaining space/word limitations as you write. Abstracts should define all non-standard abbreviations (i.e., abbreviations not considered standard by the instructions) upon first use, and use units for values as instructed (e.g. mmol/L vs. mg/dL, centimeters vs. inches, etc.).

- *Introduction/Background.* This section should be no longer than one or two sentences. It should provide essential information that allows the reader/grader to understand why your work is noteworthy. This should be specific—e.g., most people know heart failure is bad and surviving longer is good; your introduction on a study of a new aldosterone inhibitor in heart failure need not waste space on these general comments, but should focus on why your novel inhibitor may be of particular value.

- *Objective.* This section may also be termed "Hypothesis" or "Specific Aim," or may simply be included as part of your Introduction. It is applicable primarily to research abstracts, but can be used in case reports as well. Here you must answer the most fundamental question of your work: What were you trying to accomplish with this project? Why was the study done? What research question

130

were you trying to answer, or what value will you identify in this case report? This should be specific, clearly stated, and concise.

- *Methods.* For research papers, meta-analyses and systematic reviews, your Methods section must contain enough information for the readers to understand your experimental design, inclusion criteria (i.e., what subjects were studied or what published papers were included), size of the study (N, duration of follow-up, or number of papers in your review), and any specific experimental techniques employed. Also list the key statistical test(s) you used and parameters of significance (p value).

  Keeping the Methods section short is a big challenge—we all like to convey how thoughtful a study we performed, and there is a clear need to give enough information for the reviewer (or reader for abstracts introducing full manuscripts) to understand that valid experimental or selection methods were employed. One helpful technique is to review previously published/presented abstracts similar to yours—particularly those using similar experimental methods. Note how much detail these authors included (or excluded) in their Methods section, and include similar information in your abstract. Imitating success is not a bad approach to abstract writing, and to other writing endeavors as well.

- *Results.* The Results section should only address the key results that answer the questions of your hypotheses or specific aims. Give critical numbers (with standard deviations) for the primary dependent variable of your study. If the abstract is for a case report, this concept includes the key observation you made and supported with your literature review: for example, "Chest pain is absent among 52% of women suffering an acute myocardial infarction." Again, be frugal in your word usage, avoiding repetition of material from your Methods section. For example, if no significant difference was found between groups, it isn't necessary to state this *and* include a non-significant p value. Conversely, if your p value is significant, just list the p value—you will have stated your significance level previously.

Additionally, don't include results of questions not stated previously. If your Introduction (or Specific Aims) section stated your goal was to determine the frequency with which women with AMI presented without typical chest pain, don't insert additional information, such as their troponin levels or EKG findings, unless you introduced them as questions your project sought to answer. Such "post hoc" findings are at best interesting but nonetheless arbitrary findings of your project, and reviewers might conclude you were "fishing" for something positive to state, particularly if your primary hypothesis findings were negative.

Another word about graphics: A graph or table will typically take up at least half of your abstract space, so in general they are not advisable. However, some data can be presented with more detail in less space with a table, simple bar graph, or line chart. How do you know if a graphic will work in your abstract? One way is to try to write your results in text and see if you can convey what you want without a graphic. If you find, after several attempts, that this approach isn't working, create and insert your graphic, and try again. Remember to not repeat information in both graphic and text.

- *Conclusions.* The last section of your abstract is a summary statement, either the conclusions you have drawn from the work, or a "take-home message" from your case study or systematic literature review. It may include something related to the clinical applicability or impact of your findings. The goal is *one* sentence—as concise and specific as possible. Avoid overstatement but also don't be too humble (with hedging, nebulous phrases). Appropriate concluding statements might be: "Tyrosine kinase inhibition with Drug X reduces the ability of melanoma cells to adhere to endothelial cells." Statements such as "Tyrosine kinase inhibitors are the most important drugs to cure cancer" or "Tyrosine kinase inhibitors could possibly be useful adjuncts for some patients with certain types of malignancy" are not good choices. For a case and review, it might be "The diagnosis of acute myocardial infarction should not be excluded in women without ischemic chest pain upon presentation," rather than "Woman usually have silent myocardial infarctions" or "These findings could be important for physicians seeing patients in the emergency department setting."

———————◆———————

Abstract writing is more art than science, and you will improve both in the quality of your finished abstracts and your efficiency in writing quality pieces with experience. When just starting out, a few facts can save you time, effort, and perhaps avoid unnecessary rejections. Read published abstracts and take note of style, techniques, content, and detail; also note what isn't there, particularly related to detail and graphics. Like most scholarly activities, getting advice from experienced colleagues can be invaluable. Most importantly, don't be disappointed if your initial attempts at abstract writing are unsuccessful: understand that becoming an effective abstract author is a process, during which you will make mistakes; learn from them, and do better the next time.

Chapter 17
Notes on Platform Presentations

The term "Platform Presentation" is applied to a timed, oral presentation given at a regional or national professional meeting. "Platforms" are usually part of a symposium of topic-specific research or case presentations within a given discipline. The most common format is a ten-minute presentation using projected visuals (slides or cines), followed by five minutes for questions from the audience. The presentations may be held in small classrooms seating 40-50 people, or large auditoriums or lecture halls with several thousand attendees.

The common factor to all platform presentations is a strict time limitation. At larger meetings where a ten-minute limit is given for each presentation, for example, a lighting system is often employed: a green light is visible to the speaker for the first nine minutes of his or her talk; an amber light appears at the beginning of the tenth minute; a blinking red light appears with 15 seconds remaining in the ten-minute limit; and a constant red light appears when the speaker's time has expired. Moderators will usually interrupt the speaker 10-15 seconds after the red light appears. With such strict time limits, there are some principles that will help you give a successful platform presentation. These include:

Limit your primary slides. Normally a title slide (with institutional affiliations and funding disclosures), a conflict-of-interest slide (usually required), and 8-12 content slides are about all you can present comfortably in this timeframe. You can (and should) have back-up slides for the question period for any inquiries you can anticipate.

Use your abstract as an outline in preparing your slides. Remember the abstract earned you the presentation opportunity, and professional audiences expect your work to be presented in a sequence that parallels your structured abstract.

Don't try to say too much. Get the critical information out as Background, Methods, Results and Conclusions. Use graphics whenever possible. Limit the text on your slides (using outlines, bullet lists, and simple tables) and avoid text slides with full sentences (except perhaps for your conclusions). You very well may be unable to present everything you would like in ten minutes, but spend this valuable time on the most important aspects of your work.

Consider scripting your presentation. A platform presentation is the one setting where scripting can be a good idea. Time is so limited that any verbal stumbling during the presentation could leave you with insufficient opportunity to convey your conclusions. It can be helpful to write the script for each slide, inserting marks where you will point to a section on the slide, or allow a pause for the audience to take in the information. Prints of slide miniatures (used as a speaking guide) can also be helpful in keying your remarks.

Practice your presentation repeatedly. Aim to complete your talk within nine to nine-and-one-half minutes. Look for ways to convey your message with fewer words. With practice, you will be able to get through more information in a scripted presentation than simply keying off your slides, and well-prepared phrases can increase your presentation efficiency remarkably. Use time markers: one minute for introduction and background, two minutes for methods, etc. Practice (and present) with your watch or clock next to your notes. Once you think you have it down, ask colleagues and mentors to watch and critique your presentation. Sometimes having your presentation video-taped and watching yourself present can be enlightening, and you will find opportunities to polish, shorten, and emphasize what you might never have identified without such a tool. Practice is also the best treatment for anxiety.

Dress professionally. Platform presentations are a big deal: coats and ties for men; business suits for women. Casual attire has no place on the podium at most meetings.

Act professionally. Always start out by addressing the moderators and audience. This is a sign of a seasoned professional. Beginning your talk with something like "Dr. Jones, Dr. Smith, ladies and gentlemen" may sound trite but it conveys respect for your colleagues, the meeting and the organization. Also, thank the audience for their time and attention at the end. Be sure you are speaking into the microphone at all times.

Bring everything you need. Even if you have submitted your slides electronically in advance, bring two back-ups on USB drives, CD/DVDs or other portable media. Bring a laser pointer, and two printed copies of your scripted presentation. Keep the copies in different places—don't risk not having what you need.

Know your work. If there is any aspect of your presentation you could not explain to a topic novice at a high school level, go back to the books before you present. You do not know who will be in the audience, how specialized their knowledge of the field, and whether they may believe differently than the results you are presenting. Do your homework.

Don't let questions upset you. Most of the time, questions from the audience are genuine and not intended to catch you or show you up. Take your time, think, and answer as honestly as possible. If presented with a question or issue you hadn't considered, admit to this and thank the questioner for the idea. If you think a comment is hostile, and your honest responses have failed to satisfy the questioner, your options include: (1) agreeing with the questioner (no one can argue with you if you agree with them); (2) saying you may not be stating your answer clearly and will be happy to speak with him or her individually after the session (another way to quell dissent from the podium); and (3) stating you do not have the detailed answer at hand but will check your records to provide a more accurate response via email after the meeting (again, a non-confrontational approach). Above all else, don't get into an argument with an attendee: even if you win, you lose.

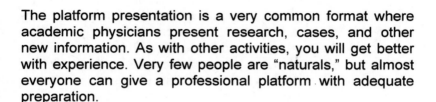

The platform presentation is a very common format where academic physicians present research, cases, and other new information. As with other activities, you will get better with experience. Very few people are "naturals," but almost everyone can give a professional platform with adequate preparation.

Chapter 18
Notes on Poster Presentations

The original purpose of poster presentations at professional meetings was to convey preliminary results of scientific studies to the interested community before hard copy publications could be printed and distributed. When compared to platform presentations, posters offered the opportunity for many presenters to have their studies viewable simultaneously, and for attendees to choose among those they considered most relevant to their interests and needs. Over time, poster sessions grew in breadth and application to include almost every type of field, topic, intent, and venue.

Academic physicians most often present posters on some type of scientific study or case report. Typically, but not always, submissions are selected through a competitive process by an organization representing professionals in a given field. For some meetings, abstracts may be submitted for general consideration—either platform or poster presentation—or specifically for poster presentation only. The competitive phase usually involves refereed grading of submitted abstracts (see Chapter 16, *Notes on Writing an Abstract*); once accepted and assigned, the sponsor will provide specific instructions on how posters are to be prepared for its meeting.

The greatest value of presenting a poster is the input you will receive from meeting attendees. Even if not required, you should be physically present at your poster venue as long as possible to answer questions and speak with the professionals who come to learn about your work.

Your Poster
As computer and printing technology continues to advance, creation of a hard-copy poster has become far easier than it was previously. Software programs, such as Microsoft PowerPoint and Adobe InDesign, make creating graphs and tables, text entries, and title panels a simple process: they allow for almost limitless re-organization of layout, right up until the actual printing. With such flexibility, however, comes

the added temptation of including too much information or ending up with a poster that is difficult to read at a distance. Attention to a few principles will help you create a professional poster that will effectively communicate your information to session attendees.

Have an effective title. Your abstract title must be your poster title, and it will be listed as such in the program (and abstract publications). You want a title that will attract interested attendees to your poster from among the dozens, or hundreds, simultaneously offered. It should be sufficiently specific to be correctly identified by attendees, but not so detailed as to make it unreadable by those walking through the presentation hall.

Avoid too many words. Attendees should be able to read your poster and understand the relevant information in a few minutes. Bullet lists, simple tables, graphs, and illustrations are very effective tools for posters, while formal paragraphs and complete sentences are best limited to your abstract. A picture really can be worth a thousand words, particularly in a crowded poster hall. Conversely, a "busy" poster will attract fewer attendees than one that is quick to read, easy to understand, and clear in the message it conveys.

Readability is more important than glitz. Use a font size large enough to be easily read from at least five-to-six feet away, and select a sans serif font such as Arial. Maximum contrast is most readable, so black text on a white background is best in a well-lighted hall. Use colors on your figures and illustrations, institutional logo, background, and perhaps to highlight a few key words. Avoid 3-D and other enhancements to fonts or graphics—remember it is your research, not your computer or graphic skills, that you are presenting to your audience; such enhancements may look nice but actually make interpretation more difficult than having simple, classical graphs and figures.

Organize your panels in a logical order. A poster should be able to stand alone, with information easily followed by readers even in your absence. Have colleagues without prior knowledge of your work view the poster before the meeting, without you present, to assure a logical flow and organization.

Follow the instructions. Be sure to read the instructions provided by the sponsor carefully before preparing your poster. Details such as dimensions, required information (including institutional affiliations of all authors, IRB or animal use committee approval, conflict of interest declarations, and funding statements), and any other meeting-specific requirements must be met—you won't be able to put up a poster that is larger than the allotted space, nor should you risk disqualification from award consideration by neglecting these simple details.

Additional points. Remember to bring push pins and perhaps a mechanical pointer. Your print shop can probably provide reduced copies ($8\frac{1}{2}$ x 11 inches) of your poster—which are occasionally required but always nice to have available to hand out at the meeting. Bring business cards with your contact information (including your email address) to distribute: your next collaborator (or employer) might just come by to view your work. Finally, put your poster up on time, at the very beginning of the allowable posting period; you don't want to miss attendees who might come by at the beginning of the session—they often don't return for a second look.

Your Presentation
At some meetings a time is set aside for live presentations, during which you and four or five other presenters will be expected to give brief (approximately five-minute) oral summaries of your work to a moderator and a group of referees or attendees. These sessions are especially common at smaller meetings, when your poster is among the finalists for an award or other competition, or when the sponsoring organization has chosen to highlight the posters with a dedicated (non-compete) time slot in the program schedule. If your session is specifically for trainees or young investiga-

tors, this may be the most critical part of the competition as final judging will likely weigh your oral presentation heavily toward final scoring.

Presentation of your poster to a group is not dissimilar to a platform presentation (see Chapter 17, *Notes on Platform Presentations*), except you will use panels on your poster rather than slides. Timing is usually less stringent, but it is always better to finish early than run long and be cut off by the moderator. Like other timed presentations, the key to success is practice, practice, practice.

Show professionalism at all times. Even if the meeting attire is more casual, dress professionally (coat and tie for men, business suit for women) for your presentation. Also, if yours is in a group of several oral presentations, ask questions of the other presenters when invited to do so—it will show the moderator you are part of the scholarly community and not there just to show off your work.

Finally, remove your poster from the board at the scheduled end of your session. Even if you are going to trash it after the meeting, you don't want to make it look like you don't care about your poster. Many departments and divisions have places for you to show your poster back home—on a hallway board or conference room—to advertise the scholarship of your group.

———————◆———————

A poster presentation is often the first opportunity young academic physicians have to present in an extramural setting. Like so many other activities, you will improve with time and experience. Ask for advice and guidance from senior colleagues and mentors, and prepare a poster worthy of the hard work you put into your research or case presentation.

About the Authors

Stephen A. Geraci is Professor and Vice Chairman of Internal Medicine at the University of Mississippi School of Medicine in Jackson. He is a *cum laude* graduate of the Penn State-Jefferson Medical College BS-MD program, and trained in internal medicine, cardiovascular diseases, critical care medicine, and clinical pharmacology. He has held academic appointments in internal medicine, cardiology, pulmonary and critical care medicine, pharmacology, hypertension, emergency medicine, clinical pharmacology, and clinical pharmacy, and served on faculty at the George Washington University, Uniformed Services University of the Health Sciences, University of Tennessee, University of Florida, and the University of Wisconsin-Madison. He has held leadership positions in many national professional organizations and institutions of higher learning, lectured across the country on a broad array of clinical, scientific and educational topics, and authored more than 100 manuscripts, abstracts, monographs, tutorials and web pages.

Dr. Geraci has trained hundreds of medical students, residents, fellows, undergraduate and graduate students, and entry- and mid-level faculty members in various health care disciplines, who have in turn earned regional and national young investigator awards, intramural scholarship recognition, and success in all areas of academic health care. They have held positions at a number of medical schools, universities and academic health centers across the United States.

Mary Jane Burton is Assistant Professor of Medicine at the University of Mississippi School of Medicine. She received her Doctorate of Medicine from the University of Mississippi Medical Center in 2001, and is board certified in Internal Medicine and Infectious Diseases. She is the Clinical Director of the HIV and Viral Hepatitis clinics at the G.V. Sonny Montgomery Veterans Affairs Medical Center in Jackson, has authored many peer-reviewed papers on Infectious Disease topics, and is a recent recipient of a career development award from the Veterans Healthcare Administration for her research in hepatitis C and herpes simplex virus type 2. Her clinical and research interests involve new paradigms for hepatitis C therapy in difficult-to-treat populations. She has received recognition for her accomplishments as a clinician, educator, investigator, and program developer.

Dr. Burton is also the mother of three school-aged children, and has personal experience in dealing with issues and solving problems associated with balancing family and child-rearing with a clinical academic career. Dr. Geraci was her Medical Service chief with her first faculty appointment in Jackson, and remains one of her career mentors. Dr. Burton has now herself become a mentor and advisor to trainees and junior faculty at her home institution. She is primary author on the chapters on *Pregnancy and Early Child Care*, and *Part-Time Faculty Positions*.

CPSIA information can be obtained at www.ICGtesting.com
Printed in the USA
LVOW11s2210231113

362582LV00001B/3/P

9 781612 330822